Preventing Childhood Obesity in Early Care and Education Programs

3rd Edition

D0897288

Selected Standards From

Caring for Our Children: National Health and Safety Performance Standards; Guidelines for Early Care and Education Programs, 4th Edition

Developed by

American Academy of Pediatrics
345 Park Blvd
Itasca, IL 60143

American Public Health Association
800 I St NW
Washington, DC 20001-3710

National Resource Center for Health and Safety in Child Care and Early Education
University of Colorado College of Nursing
13120 19th Ave
Aurora, CO 80045

Support for this project was provided by the Maternal and Child Health Bureau, Health Resources and Services Administration, US Department of Health and Human Services (Cooperative Agreement #U46MC09810).

American Academy
of Pediatrics

DEDICATED TO THE HEALTH OF ALL CHILDREN®

APHA PRESS

AN IMPRINT OF **AMERICAN PUBLIC HEALTH ASSOCIATION**

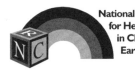

National Resource Center
for Health and Safety
in Child Care and
Early Education

Special discounts are available for bulk purchases of this publication. Email Special Sales at aapsales@aap.org for more information.

Suggested Citation:
American Academy of Pediatrics, American Public Health Association, National Resource Center for Health and Safety in Child Care and Early Education. *Preventing Childhood Obesity in Early Care and Education Programs.* 3rd ed. Itasca, IL: American Academy of Pediatrics; 2020

Printed in the United States of America

9-431   1 2 3 4 5 6 7 8 9 10

MA0937

ISBN: 978-1-61002-356-6
eBook: 978-1-61002-357-3
Cover and publication design by Linda Diamond

Library of Congress Control Number: 2018914657

CONTENTS

FOREWORD

The third edition of *Preventing Childhood Obesity in Early Care and Education Programs* (*PCO3*) is a compilation of evidence-based nutrition, physical activity, and screen time best practices in the standards published in *Caring for Our Children: National Health and Safety Performance Standards; Guidelines for Early Care and Education Programs* (http://nrckids.org/CFOC) as of April 1, 2019. *Preventing Childhood Obesity* is intended to assist early care and education programs with the development and implementation of best practices, procedures, and policies to instill healthy behaviors and lifestyle choices in young children, supporting obesity prevention.

Changes from the previous edition (2012) reflect

- Nutrition information based on the 2017 revisions to the Child and Adult Care Food Program Meal Pattern
- The current *Physical Activity Guidelines for Americans* (2018) from the US Department of Health and Human Services
- Policy changes regarding screen time and digital media use

Special thanks are due to Danette Glassy, MD, FAAP, and Christopher Bolling, MD, FAAP, chair, Executive Committee, American Academy of Pediatrics Section on Obesity, for their contribution in reviewing *PCO3* introductions and the Executive Summary. The updates to the third edition build on the effort put forth in 2010 by Nutrition Technical Panel Chair Catherine Cowell, PhD, and Technical Panel members in supporting the development of the first edition of *PCO*.

Nutrition Technical Panel Members, 2010

Catherine Cowell, PhD (Chair)
Donna Blum-Kemelor, MS, RD, LD
Robin Brocato, MHS
Kristen Copeland, MD, FAAP
Suzanne Haydu, MPH, RD
Janet Hill, MS, RD, IBCLC
Susan L. Johnson, PhD
Ruby Natale, PhD, PsyD
Sara Benjamin Neelon, PhD, MPH, RD
Jeanette Panchula, BSW, RN, PHN, IBCLC
Shana Patterson, RD
Barbara Polhamus, PhD, MPH, RD
Susan Schlosser, MS, RD
Denise Sofka, MPH, RD
Jamie Stang, PhD, MPH, RD

EXECUTIVE SUMMARY

STANDARDS ON NUTRITION, PHYSICAL ACTIVITY, AND SCREEN TIME

Research and recommended best practices link eating nutritious food, engaging in daily age-appropriate physical activities, and limiting screen time and digital media use to maintaining a child's healthy weight.[1,2] *Preventing Childhood Obesity in Early Care and Education Programs,* 3rd Edition (*PCO3*), is a set of standards from the *Caring for Our Children (CFOC) Online Standards Database.*[3] The *CFOC* online database is the most up-to-date source of early care and education health and safety standards based on scientific evidence and expert consensus. The *CFOC* standards are a leading resource for creating model policies and effective practices to promote a child's well-being in out-of-home care.

The selection of standards on nutrition, physical activity, and screen time/digital media in *PCO3* may enable early care and education programs to support healthy lifestyles for children and families, because early care and education caregivers/teachers are in a unique position to influence development of healthy eating and active habits that prevent childhood obesity.[4,5] *Preventing Childhood Obesity* standards contain practical strategies to prevent excessive weight gain in young children. These standards identify and detail opportunities for program staff to work with families by supporting breastfeeding mothers; serving fruits, vegetables, and other healthy foods; promoting daily physical activity for children of all ages; and using screen time/digital media minimally and wisely. The standards also encourage active engagement of caregivers/teachers to model healthy habits in their interactions with children.

CONTENTS

Preventing Childhood Obesity in Early Care and Education Programs includes standards in 2 topic areas: nutrition and physical activity/screen time.

- **Nutrition Standards**

  - General Requirements: Feeding Plans; Use of US Department of Agriculture Child and Adult Care Food Program Guidelines; Written Menus; Availability of Drinking Water and 100% Fruit Juice; Care of Children with Food Allergies; Vegetarian/Vegan Diets

  - Requirements for Infants: Breastfeeding; Feeding Infants on Cue by a Consistent Caregiver/Teacher; Preparing, Feeding, and Storing Human Milk or Infant Formula; Techniques for Bottle Feeding; Introduction of Age-Appropriate Solid Foods; Use of Soy-Based Formula and Soy Milk

  - Requirements for Toddlers and Preschoolers: Meal and Snack Patterns; Serving Size; Encouraging Self-Feeding; Feeding Cow's Milk

  - Requirements for School-Age Children: Meal and Snack Patterns

  - Meal Service and Supervision: Socialization During Meals; Numbers of Children Fed Simultaneously by One Adult; Adult Supervision; Experience with Familiar and New Foods; Use of Nutritionist/Registered Dietitian

  - Food Brought From Home: Nutritional Quality; Selection and Preparation

  - Nutrition Education: Nutrition Learning Experiences for Children; Nutrition Education for Parents/Guardians; Health, Nutrition, Physical Activity, and Safety Awareness

  - Policies: Food and Nutrition Service Policies and Plans; Infant Feeding Policy

- **Physical Activity/Screen Time Standards**

  - Physical Activity: Active Opportunities for Physical Activity; Playing Outdoors; Protection from Air Pollution; Caregivers'/Teachers' Encouragement of Physical Activity; Policies and Practices that Promote Physical Activity

  - Screen Time: Screen Time/Digital Media Use

SUGGESTED USES OF STANDARDS FOR PREVENTING CHILDHOOD OBESITY

- **Families** can evaluate the obesity prevention practices in their child's early care and education program. They can join caregivers/teachers in planning programs to prevent childhood obesity and encourage healthy living. Families may also want to incorporate some of these same strategies and practices at home.
- **Caregivers/teachers** can develop practices, policies, and staff training to ensure children's programs include healthy, age-appropriate feeding; abundant physical activity; and limited screen time/digital media use.
- **Health care professionals** can promote healthy weight practices by assisting families and caregivers/teachers to support age-appropriate nutrition and to encourage active playtime and limited screen time/digital media use.
- **Licensing professionals/regulators** can develop regulations based on evidence and best practices to support the prevention of obesity and promote healthy weight practices.
- **Early childhood systems** can build integrated nutrition and physical activity components into their systems that promote healthy lifestyles for all children.
- **Policy makers** are equipped with evidence and best practices to address emerging challenges to the development of lifelong healthy behavior and lifestyles.
- **Faculty** of university/college early childhood education programs can instill in their curricula healthy weight practices for students to implement on entering the early childhood workplace.

PUBLISHERS: American Academy of Pediatrics, American Public Health Association, National Resource Center for Health and Safety in Child Care and Early Education

References

1. Institute of Medicine. *Preventing Childhood Obesity: Health in the Balance.* Washington, DC: National Academies Press; 2005. https://doi.org/10.17226/11015. Accessed April 25, 2019
2. Sallis JF, Glanz K. Physical activity and food environments: solutions to the obesity epidemic. *Milbank Q.* 2009;87(1):123–154 PMID: 19298418 https://doi.org/10.1111/j.1468-0009.2009.00550.x
3. American Academy of Pediatrics, American Public Health Association, National Resource Center for Health and Safety in Child Care and Early Education. *CFOC Online Standards Database.* http://nrckids.org/CFOC. Accessed April 25, 2019
4. Story M, Kaphingst KM, French S. The role of child care settings in obesity prevention. *Future Child.* 2006;16(1):143–168 PMID: 16532662 http://www.jstor.org/stable/3556554
5. Larson N, Ward DS, Neelon SB, Story M. What role can child-care settings play in obesity prevention? A review of the evidence and call for research efforts. *J Am Diet Assoc.* 2011;111(9):1343–1362 PMID: 21872698 http://doi.org/10.1016/j.jada.2011.06.007

NUTRITION STANDARDS

Introduction

One of the basic responsibilities of every parent/guardian and caregiver/teacher is to provide nourishing food daily that is clean, safe, and developmentally appropriate for infants and children. Food is essential in any early care and education setting to keep infants and children free from hunger. Children also need freely available, clean drinking water offered throughout the day. Feeding should occur in a relaxed and pleasant environment that fosters healthy digestion and positive social behavior. Food provides energy and nutrients needed by infants and children during the critical period of their growth and development.

Feeding nutritious food everyday must be accompanied by offering appropriate daily physical activity and playtime for the healthy physical, social, and emotional development of infants and young children. There is solid evidence that physical activity can prevent a rapid gain in weight that could lead to childhood obesity early in life. The early care and education setting is an ideal environment to foster the goal of providing supervised, age-appropriate physical activity during the critical years of growth when health habits and patterns are being developed for life. The overall benefits of practicing healthy eating patterns, while being physically active daily, are significant. Physical, social, and emotional habits are developed during the early years and continue into adulthood; thus, these habits can be improved in early childhood to prevent and reduce obesity and a range of chronic diseases. Active play and supervised structured physical activities promote healthy weight; improved overall fitness, including mental health; improved bone development and cardiovascular health; and development of social skills.

Breastfeeding sets the stage for an infant to establish healthy attachment. The American Academy of Pediatrics, the US Breastfeeding Committee, the Academy of Breastfeeding Medicine, the American Academy of Family Physicians, the World Health Organization, and the United Nations Children's Fund (UNICEF) all recommend that women should breastfeed exclusively for about the first 6 months of the infant's life, adding age-appropriate solid foods (complementary foods) and continuing breastfeeding for at least the first year, if not longer.[1]

Human (breast) milk, containing all the nutrients to promote optimal growth, is the most developmentally appropriate food for infants. It changes during the course of each feeding and over time to meet the growing infant's or child's changing nutritional needs. All caregivers/teachers should be trained to encourage, support, and accommodate breastfeeding. Caregivers/teachers have a unique opportunity to support breastfeeding mothers, who are often daunted by the prospect of continuing to breastfeed as they return to work.[2] Early care and education programs can reduce a breastfeeding mother's anxiety by welcoming breastfeeding families and providing a staff that is well trained in the proper handling of human milk and feeding of breastfed infants and accommodating mothers who wish to breastfeed on site. Even when infant formula is used to supplement breast milk, the program staff should encourage the mother to continue to breastfeed and pump to avoid a decrease in breast milk production.[3]

Some families choose to feed their baby infant formula, and some infants require a special formula for a specific nutritional need. A primary health care professional should give the early care and education program a written prescription when a special infant formula is used.[4]

Given adequate opportunity, assistance, and developmentally appropriate equipment, infants learn to self-feed as age-appropriate solid foods are introduced. Infants must attain typical physical growth, motor coordination, and cognitive and social skills to learn to feed themselves. Modeling healthy eating by early care and education staff encourages a child to develop healthy eating habits.[5] At about 6 months of age, infants are more interactive with their environments and becoming more independent in their abilities to select different kinds and combinations of foods offered.

To ensure programs are offering a variety of foods, selections should be made from the following groups of food[4]:

a. Fruits
b. Vegetables
c. Whole grains
d. Protein
e. Dairy

Current research recommends a diet rich in essential nutrients, including protein, carbohydrates, healthy fats, vitamins, and minerals with sufficient calories to meet the child's needs. The availability of a variety of clean, safe, nourishing foods is essential to foster periods of rapid growth and development.

As part of their developing growth and maturity, toddlers often exhibit new and sometimes erratic eating habits. One child may want to eat the same food for several days or weeks, while another may become a picky eater, dawdling or refusing to eat certain foods. Introduction of new foods may become challenging due to new tastes, colors, odors, or textures. If eating patterns become problematic (eg, failure to thrive, excessive weight gains), parents/guardians, caregivers/teachers, and the primary health care professional should collaborate on a plan to address the issue. Consistent implementation of the plan is important to help a child to build sound eating habits. Family homes and center-based out-of-home early care and education settings have the opportunity to guide and support children's sound eating habits and food learning experiences.[6]

Attitudes about food and eating behaviors are formed at an early age. For example, response to infant and child cues for hunger helps to foster trust and reduces overfeeding and overeating. Healthy food habits are built by eating and enjoying a variety of nutritious foods that may also include families' cultural preferences.[7] A balanced diet, combined with daily age-appropriate physical activity, can reduce the risk of overweight, obesity, and chronic disease in children later in life.[8–10]

The following nutrition and food service standards, along with related appendixes (eg, the US Department of Agriculture MyPlate) and other resources (eg, *2015–2020 Dietary Guidelines for Americans*), address age-appropriate foods and feeding techniques beginning with the very first food and continuing throughout the early years.

REFERENCES

1. Azad MB, Vehling L, Chan D, et al; CHILD Study Investigators. Infant feeding and weight gain: separating breast milk from breastfeeding and formula from food. *Pediatrics.* 2018;142(4):e20181092 PMID: 30249624 http://doi.org/10.1542/peds.2018-1092

2. Calloway EE, Stern KL, Schober DJ, Yaroch AL. Creating supportive breastfeeding policies in early childhood education programs: a qualitative study from a multi-site intervention. *Matern Child Health J.* 2017;21(4):809–817 PMID: 27520557 https://doi.org/10.1007/s10995-016-2174-y

3. US Department of Health and Human Services. *The Surgeon General's Call to Action to Support Breastfeeding.* Washington, DC: US Department of Health and Human Services, Office of the Surgeon General; 2011. https://www.surgeongeneral.gov/library/calls/breastfeeding/calltoactiontosupportbreastfeeding.pdf. Accessed April 25, 2019

4. US Department of Agriculture Food and Nutrition Service. Child and Adult Care Food Program (CACFP). https://www.fns.usda.gov/cacfp/child-and-adult-care-food-program. Published August 6, 2018. Accessed April 25, 2019

5. Cotwright CJ, Bales DW, Lee JS, Parrott K, Celestin N, Olubajo B. Like peas and carrots: combining wellness policy implementation with classroom education for obesity prevention in the childcare setting. *Public Health Rep.* 2017;132(2 suppl):74S–80S PMID: 29136489 https://doi.org/10.1177/0033354917719706

6. American Academy of Pediatrics Committee on Nutrition. *Pediatric Nutrition.* Kleinman RE, Greer FR, eds. 7th ed. Elk Grove Village, IL: American Academy of Pediatrics; 2014

7. US Department of Agriculture. ChooseMyPlate.gov. Healthy eating style. https://www.choosemyplate.gov/healthy-eating-style. Updated October 12, 2016. Accessed April 25, 2019

8. US Department of Health and Human Services, US Department of Agriculture. *2015–2020 Dietary Guidelines for Americans.* 8th ed. Washington, DC: US Government Printing Office; 2015. https://health.gov/dietaryguidelines/2015/resources/2015-2020_Dietary_Guidelines.pdf. Accessed April 25, 2019

9. US Department of Health and Human Services. *Physical Activity Guidelines for Americans.* 2nd ed. Washington, DC: US Department of Health and Human Services; 2018. https://health.gov/paguidelines/second-edition/pdf/Physical_Activity_Guidelines_2nd_edition.pdf. Accessed April 25, 2019

10. Lindsay AC, Greaney ML, Wallington SF, Mesa T, Salas CF. A review of early influences on physical activity and sedentary behaviors of preschool-age children in high-income countries. *J Spec Pediatr Nurs.* 2017;22(3):e12182 PMID: 28407367 https://doi.org/10.1111/jspn.12182

General Requirements

Written Nutrition Plan

The facility should provide nourishing and appealing food for children according to a written plan developed by a qualified nutritionist/registered dietitian. Caregivers/teachers, directors, and food service personnel should share the responsibility for carrying out the plan. The director is responsible for implementing the plan but may delegate tasks to caregivers/teachers and food service personnel.

Where infants and young children are involved, the feeding plan may include special attention to supporting mothers in maintaining their human milk supply. The nutrition plan should include steps to take when problems require rapid response by the staff, such as when a child chokes during mealtime or has an allergic reaction to a food. The completed plan should be on file, easily accessible to staff, and available to parents/guardians on request.

If the facility is large enough to justify employment of a full-time nutritionist/registered dietitian or child care food service manager, the facility should delegate to this person the responsibility for implementing the written plan. Some children may have medical conditions that require special dietary modifications. A written care plan from the primary health care provider, clearly stating the food(s) to be avoided and food(s) to be substituted, should be on file.

This information should be updated annually if the modification is not a lifetime special dietary need. Staff should be educated about a child's dietary modification to ensure that no child in care ingests or has contact with foods he/she should avoid while at the facility. The proper modifications should be implemented whether the child brings his/her own food or whether it is prepared on site. The facility needs to inform all families and staff if certain foods, such as nut products (e.g., peanut butter, peanut oil), should not be brought from home because of a child's life-threatening allergy. Staff should also know what procedure to follow if ingestion or contact occurs. In addition to knowing ahead of time what procedures to follow, staff must know their designated roles during an emergency. The emergency plan should be dated and updated biannually.

RATIONALE

Nourishing and appealing food is the cornerstone of children's health, growth, and development, as well as developmentally appropriate learning experiences (1–3). Nutrition and feeding are fundamental and required in every facility. Because children grow and develop more rapidly during the first few years after birth than at any other time, a child's home and the facility together must provide food that is adequate in amount and type to meet each child's growth and nutritional needs. Children can learn healthy eating habits and be better equipped to maintain a healthy weight if they eat nourishing food while attending early care and education settings (4). Children can self-regulate their food intake and are able to determine an appropriate amount of food to eat in any one sitting when allowed to feed themselves. Excessive

prompting, feeding in response to emotional distress, and using food as a reward have all been shown to lead to excessive weight gain in children (5,6). The obesity epidemic makes this an important lesson today.

Meals and snacks provide the caregiver/teacher an opportunity to model appropriate mealtime behavior and guide the conversation, which aids in children's conceptual and sensory language development and eye/hand coordination. In larger facilities, professional nutrition staff must be involved to ensure compliance with nutrition and food service guidelines, including accommodation of children with special health care needs.

RELATED STANDARDS

Assessment and Planning of Nutrition for Individual Children
Categories of Foods
Feeding Plans and Dietary Modifications
Feeding Infants on Cue by a Consistent Caregiver/Teacher
Use of Nutritionist/Registered Dietitian
Prohibited Uses of Food
Nutrition Learning Experiences for Children
Food and Nutrition Service Policies and Plans
Appendix: Nutrition Specialist, Registered Dietitian, Licensed
  Nutritionist, Consultant, and Food Service Staff Qualifications

REFERENCES

1. US Department of Health and Human Services, Administration for Children and Families, Office of Head Start. *Head Start Program Performance Standards.* Rev ed. Washington, DC: US Government Printing Office; 2016. https://eclkc.ohs.acf.hhs.gov/policy/45-cfr-chap-xiii. Accessed September 7, 2017
2. Hagan JF, Shaw JS, Duncan PM, eds. *Bright Futures: Guidelines for Health Supervision of Infants, Children, and Adolescents.* 4th ed. Elk Grove Village, IL: American Academy of Pediatrics; 2017
3. Holt K, Wooldridge N, Story M, Sofka D. *Bright Futures: Nutrition.* 3rd ed. Elk Grove Village, IL: American Academy of Pediatrics; 2011
4. Kleinman RE, Greer FR, eds. *Pediatric Nutrition.* 7th ed. Elk Grove Village, IL: American Academy of Pediatrics; 2014
5. Lally JR, Griffin A, Fenichel E, Segal M, Szanton E, Weissbourd B. *Caring for Infants and Toddlers in Groups: Developmentally Appropriate Practice.* 2nd ed. Arlington, VA: Zero to Three; 2008

NOTES
Content in the STANDARD was modified on 11/9/2017.

Routine Health Supervision and Growth Monitoring

The facility should require that each child has routine health supervision by the child's primary care provider, according to the standards of the American Academy of Pediatrics (AAP) (3). For all children, health supervision includes routine screening tests, immunizations, and chronic or acute illness monitoring. For children younger than twenty-four months of age, health supervision includes documentation and plotting of sex-specific charts on child growth standards from the World Health Organization (WHO), available at http://www.who.int/childgrowth/standards/en/, and assessing diet and activity. For children twenty-four months of age and older, sex-specific height and weight graphs should be plotted by the primary care provider in addition to body mass index (BMI), according to the Centers for Disease Control and Prevention (CDC). BMI is classified as underweight (BMI less than 5%), healthy weight (BMI 5%–84%), overweight (BMI 85%–94%), and obese (BMI equal to or greater than 95%). Follow-up visits with the child's primary care provider that include a full assessment and laboratory evaluations should be scheduled for children with weight for length greater than 95% and BMI greater than 85% (5).

School health services can meet this standard for school-age children in care if they meet the AAP's standards for school-age children and if the results of each child's examinations are shared with the caregiver/teacher as well as with the school health system. With parental/guardian consent, pertinent health information should be exchanged among the child's routine source of health care and all participants in the child's care, including any school health program involved in the care of the child.

RATIONALE
Provision of routine preventive health services for children ensures healthy growth and development and helps detect disease when it is most treatable. Immunization prevents or reduces diseases for which effective vaccines are available. When children are receiving care that involves the school health system, such care should be coordinated by the exchange of information, with parental/guardian permission, among the school health system, the child's medical home, and the caregiver/teacher. Such exchange will ensure that all participants in the child's care are aware of the child's health status and follow a common care plan. The plotting of height and weight measurements and plotting and classification of BMI by the primary care provider or school health personnel, on a reference growth chart, will show how children are growing over time and how they compare with other children of the same chronological age and sex (1,3,4). Growth charts are based on data from national probability samples, representative of children in the general population. Their use by the primary care provider may facilitate early

recognition of growth concerns, leading to further evaluation, diagnosis, and the development of a plan of care. Such a plan of care, if communicated to the caregiver/teacher, can direct the caregiver's/teacher's attention to disease, poor nutrition, or inadequate physical activity that requires modification of feeding or other health practices in the early care and education setting (2).

COMMENTS
Periodic and accurate height and weight measurements that are obtained, plotted, and interpreted by a person who is competent in performing these tasks provide an important indicator of health status. If such measurements are made in the early care and education facility, the data from the measurements should be shared by the facility, subject to parental/guardian consent, with everyone involved in the child's care, including parents/guardians, caregivers/teachers, and the child's primary care provider. The child care health consultant can provide staff training on growth assessment. It is important to maintain strong linkage among the early care and education facility, school, parent/guardian, and the child's primary care provider. Screening results (physical and behavioral) and laboratory assessments are only useful if a plan for care can be developed to initiate and maintain lifestyle changes that incorporate the child's activities during their time at the early care and education program.

The Special Supplemental Nutrition Program for Women, Infants, and Children (WIC) can also be a source for the BMI data with parental/guardian consent, as WIC tracks growth and development if the child is enrolled.

For BMI charts by sex and age, see http://www.cdc.gov/growthcharts/clinical_charts.htm.

RELATED STANDARD
Assessment and Planning of Nutrition for Individual Children

REFERENCES
1. Paige, D. M. 1988. *Clinical nutrition*. 2nd ed. St. Louis: Mosby.
2. Kleinman, R. E. 2009. *Pediatric nutrition handbook*. 6th ed. Elk Grove Village, IL: American Academy of Pediatrics.
3. Hagan, J. F., J. S. Shaw, P. M. Duncan, eds. 2008. *Bright futures: Guidelines for health supervision of infants, children, and adolescents*. 3rd ed. Elk Grove Village, IL: American Academy of Pediatrics.
4. Story, M., K. Holt, D. Sofka, eds. 2002. *Bright futures in practice: Nutrition*. 2nd ed. Arlington, VA: National Center for Education in Maternal and Child Health.
5. Centers for Disease Control and Prevention. 2011. About BMI for children and teens. http://www.cdc.gov/healthyweight/assessing/bmi/childrens_bmi/about_childrens_bmi.html.

Assessment and Planning of Nutrition for Individual Children

As a part of routine health supervision by a primary health care provider, children should be evaluated for nutrition-related medical problems, such as failure to thrive, overweight, obesity, food allergy, reflux disease, and iron-deficiency anemia (1). The nutritional standards throughout this document are general recommendations that may not always be appropriate for some children with medically identified special nutrition needs. Caregivers/teachers should communicate with the child's parent/guardian and pediatrician/other physician to adapt nutritional offerings to individual children as indicated and medically appropriate. Caregivers/teachers should work with the parent/guardian to implement individualized feeding plans developed by the child's primary health care provider to meet a child's unique nutritional needs.

These plans could include, for instance, additional iron-rich foods for a child who has been diagnosed as having iron-deficiency anemia. For a child diagnosed as obese or overweight, the plan would focus on controlling portion sizes and creating a menu plan in which calorie-dense foods, like sugar-sweetened juices, nectars, and beverages, should not be served. Using these nutritional differences as educational moments will help children understand why they can or cannot eat certain food items. Some children require special feeding techniques, such as thickened foods or special positioning during meals. Other children will require dietary modifications based on food intolerances, such as lactose or wheat (gluten) intolerance. Some children will need dietary modifications based on cultural or religious preferences, such as vegan, vegetarian, or kosher diets, or halal foods.

RATIONALE

The early years are a critical time for children's growth and development. Nutritional problems must be identified and treated during this period to prevent serious or long-term medical problems. Strong evidence shows a relationship between preschool-aged children being presented with larger sized portions and increased energy intake, prompting the importance of implementing proper portion sizing as soon as 2 years of age for children at risk of being overweight (2). The early care and education setting may be offering most of a child's daily nutritional intake, especially for children in full-time care. It is important that the facility ensures that food offerings are congruent with nutritional interventions or dietary modifications recommended by the child's pediatrician/other physician, in consultation with the nutritionist/registered dietitian, to make certain the intervention is child specific.

RELATED STANDARDS
Routine Health Supervision and Growth Monitoring
Feeding Plans and Dietary Modifications
Feeding Infants on Cue by a Consistent Caregiver/Teacher

REFERENCES
1. McAllister JW. *Achieving a Shared Plan of Care with Children and Youth with Special Health Care Needs.* Palo Alto, CA: Lucille Packard Foundation for Children's Health; 2014. http://www.lpfch.org/sites/default/files/field/publications/achieving_a_shared_plan_of_care_full.pdf. Accessed September 7, 2017
2. McCrickerd K, Leong C, Forde CG. Preschool children's sensitivity to teacher-served portion size is linked to age related differences in leftovers. *Appetite.* 2017;114:320–328

ADDITIONAL RESOURCE
US Department of Health and Human Services, US Department of Agriculture. *2015—2020 Dietary Guidelines for Americans.* 8th ed. Washington, DC: US Department of Health and Human Services; 2015. https://health.gov/dietaryguidelines/2015/resources/2015-2020_Dietary_Guidelines.pdf. Accessed September 7, 2017

NOTES
Content in the STANDARD was modified on 11/9/2017.

Feeding Plans and Dietary Modifications

Before a child enters an early care and education facility, the facility should obtain a written history that contains any special nutrition or feeding needs for the child, including use of human milk or any special feeding utensils. The staff should review this history with the child's parents/guardians, clarifying and discussing how the parents'/guardians' home feeding routines may differ from the facility's planned routine. The child's primary health care provider should provide written information to the parent/guardian about any dietary modifications or special feeding techniques that are required at the early care and education program so they can be shared with and implemented by the program.

If dietary modifications are indicated, based on a child's medical or special dietary needs, caregivers/teachers should modify or supplement the child's diet to meet the individual child's specific needs. Dietary modifications should be made in consultation with the parents/guardians and the child's primary health care provider. Caregivers/teachers can consult with a nutritionist/registered dietitian.

A child's diet may be modified because of food sensitivity, a food allergy, or many other reasons. Food sensitivity includes a range of conditions in which a child exhibits an adverse reaction to a food that, in some instances, can be life-threatening. Modification of a child's diet may also be related to a food allergy, an inability to digest or to tolerate certain foods, a need for extra calories, a need for special positioning while eating, diabetes and the need to match food with insulin, food idiosyncrasies, and other identified feeding issues, including celiac disease, phenylketonuria, diabetes, and severe food allergy (anaphylaxis). In some cases, a child may become ill if he/she is unable to eat, so missing a meal could have a negative consequence, especially for children with diabetes.

For a child with special health care needs who requires dietary modifications or special feeding techniques, written instructions from the child's parent/guardian and the child's primary health care provider should be provided in the child's record and carried out accordingly. Dietary modifications should be recorded. These written instructions must identify

a. The child's full name and date of instructions
b. The child's special health care needs
c. Any dietary restrictions based on those special needs
d. Any special feeding or eating utensils
e. Any foods to be omitted from the diet and any foods to be substituted
f. Any other pertinent information about the child's special health care needs
g. What, if anything, needs to be done if the child is exposed to restricted foods

The written history of special nutrition or feeding needs should be used to develop individual feeding plans and, collectively, to develop facility menus. Health care providers with experience in disciplines related to special nutrition needs, including nutrition, nursing, speech therapy, occupational therapy, and physical therapy, should participate when needed and/or when they are available to the facility. If available, the nutritionist/registered dietitian should approve menus that accommodate needed dietary modifications.

The feeding plan should include steps to take when a situation arises that requires rapid response by the staff, such as a child choking during mealtime or a child with a known history of food allergies demonstrating signs and symptoms of anaphylaxis (severe allergic reaction), such as difficulty breathing and severe redness and swelling of the face or mouth. The completed plan should be on file and accessible to staff and available to parents/guardians on request.

RATIONALE

Children with special health care needs may have individual requirements related to diet and swallowing, involving special feeding utensils and feeding needs that will necessitate the development of an individual plan prior to their entry into the facility (1). Many children with special health care needs have difficulty with feeding, including delayed attainment of basic chewing, swallowing, and independent feeding skills. Food, eating style, food utensils, and equipment, including furniture, may have to be adapted to meet the developmental and physical needs of individual children (2,3).

Some children have difficulty with slow weight gain and need their caloric intake monitored and supplemented. Others, such as those with diabetes, may need to have their diet matched to their medication (e.g., insulin, if they are on a fixed dose of insulin). Some children are unable to tolerate certain foods because of their allergy to the food or their inability to digest it. The 8 most common foods to cause anaphylaxis in children are cow's milk, eggs, soy, wheat, fish, shellfish, peanuts, and tree nuts (3). Staff members must know ahead of time what procedures to follow, as well as their designated roles, during an emergency.

As a safety and health precaution, staff should know in advance whether a child has food allergies, inborn errors of metabolism, diabetes, celiac disease, tongue thrust, or special health care needs related to feeding, such as requiring special feeding utensils or equipment, nasogastric or gastric tube feedings, or special positioning. These situations require individual planning prior to the child's entry into an early care and education program and on an ongoing basis (2).

In some cases, dietary modifications are based on religious or cultural beliefs. Detailed information on each child's special needs, whether stemming from dietary, feeding equipment, or cultural needs, is invaluable to the facility staff in meeting the nutritional needs of all the children in their care.

COMMENTS

Close collaboration between families and the facility is necessary for children on special diets. Parents/guardians may have to provide food on a temporary, or even permanent, basis, if the facility, after exploring all community resources, is unable to provide the special diet.

Programs may consider using the American Academy of Pediatrics (AAP) Allergy and Anaphylaxis Emergency Plan, which is included in the AAP clinical report, Guidance on Completing a Written Allergy and Anaphylaxis Emergency Plan (4).

RELATED STANDARDS
Written Nutrition Plan
Assessment and Planning of Nutrition for Individual Children
Vegetarian/Vegan Diets
Feeding Infants on Cue by a Consistent Caregiver/Teacher

REFERENCES

1. Samour PQ, King K. *Pediatric Nutrition*. 4th ed. Sunbury, MA: Jones and Bartlett Learning; 2010
2. Kleinman RE, Greer FR, eds. *Pediatric Nutrition*. 7th ed. Elk Grove Village, IL: American Academy of Pediatrics; 2014
3. Kaczkowski CH, Caffrey C. Pediatric nutrition. In: Blanchfield DS, ed. *The Gale Encyclopedia of Children's Health: Infancy Through Adolescence*. Vol 3. 3rd ed. Farmington Hills, MI: Gale; 2016:2063–2066
4. Wang J, Sicherer SH; American Academy of Pediatrics Section on Allergy and Immunology. Guidance on completing a written allergy and anaphylaxis emergency plan. *Pediatrics*. 2017;139(3):e20164005

NOTES
Content in the STANDARD was modified on 11/9/2017.

Use of US Department of Agriculture Child and Adult Care Food Program Guidelines

All meals and snacks and their preparation, service, and storage should meet the requirements for meals (7 CFR §226.20) of the child care component of the US Department of Agriculture Child and Adult Care Food Program (CACFP) (1–3).

RATIONALE
The CACFP regulations, policies, and guidance materials on meal requirements provide basic guidelines for sound nutrition and sanitation practices. The CACFP guidance for meals and snack patterns ensures that the nutritional needs of infants and children, including school-aged children through 12 years, are met based on the Dietary Guidelines for Americans (4,5) as well as other evidence-based recommendations (6,7). Programs not eligible for reimbursement under the regulations of CACFP should still use the CACFP food guidance.

COMMENTS
Staff should use information about the child's growth and CACFP meal patterns to develop individual feeding plans (6).

RELATED STANDARDS
Routine Health Supervision and Growth Monitoring
Categories of Foods
Meal and Snack Patterns
Feeding Infants on Cue by a Consistent Caregiver/Teacher
Meal and Snack Patterns for Toddlers and Preschoolers
Meal and Snack Patterns for School-Age Children

REFERENCES

1. US Department of Agriculture, Food and Nutrition Service. Requirements for meals. US Government Publishing Office Web site. https://www.ecfr. gov/cgi-bin/text-idx?SID=9c3a6681dbf6 aada3632967c4bfeb030&mc=true&node=pt7.4.226&rgn=div5 #se7.4.226_120. Accessed September 7, 2017
2. US Department of Agriculture, Food and Nutrition Service. Child and Adult Care Food Program (CACFP). Regulations. https://www.fns. usda.gov/cacfp/regulations. Updated September 7, 2017. Accessed September 7, 2017
3. Lally JR, Griffin A, Fenichel E, Segal M, Szanton E, Weissbourd B. *Caring for Infants and Toddlers in Groups: Developmentally Appropriate Practice*. 2nd ed. Arlington, VA: Zero to Three; 2008
4. US Department of Agriculture, Food and Nutrition Service. *Independent Child Care Centers: A Child and Adult Care Food Program Handbook*. Washington, DC: US Department of Agriculture; 2014. https://fns-prod. azureedge.net/sites/default/files/cacfp/ Independent%20Child%20Care%20 Centers%20Handbook.pdf. Accessed September 7, 2017
5. US Department of Health and Human Services, US Department of Agriculture. *2015–2020 Dietary Guidelines for Americans*. 8th ed. Washington, DC: US Department of Health and Human Services; 2015. https://health.gov/dietaryguidelines/2015/resources/2015-2020_ Dietary_ Guidelines.pdf. Accessed September 7, 2017
6. US Department of Agriculture, Food and Nutrition Service. Child and Adult Food Program (CACFP). Nutrition standards for CACFP meals and snacks. https://www.fns.usda.gov/cacfp/meals-and-snacks. Updated March 27, 2017. Accessed September 7, 2017
7. US Department of Agriculture, Healthy Meals Resource System, Team Nutrition. CACFP wellness resources for child care providers. https://healthymeals.fns.usda.gov/cacfp-wellness-resources-child-care-providers. Accessed September 7, 2017

ADDITIONAL RESOURCE
US Department of Agriculture. Child and Adult Care Food Program: best practices. US Department of Agriculture, Food and Nutrition Service Web site. https://www.fns.usda.gov/sites/default/files/cacfp/CACFP_factBP. pdf. Accessed September 7, 2017

NOTES
Content in the STANDARD was modified on 11/9/2017.

Categories of Foods

The early care and education program should ensure the following food groups are being served to children in care. When incorporated into a child's diet, these food groups make up foundational components of a healthy eating pattern.

OTHER RECOMMENDATIONS

- Trans-fatty acids (trans fat) should be avoided.
- Avoid concentrated sweets such as candy, sodas, sweetened caffeinated drinks, fruit nectars, and flavored milks. Offer foods that have little or no added sugars.
- Limit salty foods such as chips and pretzels. When buying foods, choose no salt added, low-sodium, or reduced sodium versions, and prepare foods without adding salt. Use herbs or no-salt spice mixes instead of salt, soy sauce, ketchup, barbeque sauce, pickles, olives, salad dressings, butter, stick margarine, gravy, or cream sauce with seasonal vegetables and other dishes.
- Avoid caffeine.

ADDITIONAL RESOURCES

American Academy of Pediatrics. American Academy of Pediatrics recommends no fruit juice for children under 1 year. https://www.aap.org/en-us/about-the-aap/aap-press-room/Pages/American-Academy-of-Pediatrics-Recommends-No-Fruit-Juice-For-Children-Under-1-Year.aspx. Published May 22, 2017. Accessed September 19, 2017

Holt K, Wooldridge N, Story M, Sofka D. *Bright Futures: Nutrition*. 3rd ed. Elk Grove Village, IL: American Academy of Pediatrics; 2011

US Department of Agriculture. ChooseMyPlate.gov. Children. http://www.choosemyplate.gov/children. Updated August 26, 2015. Accessed September 19, 2017

US Department of Health and Human Services. *2008 Physical Activity Guidelines for Americans*. Washington, DC: US Department of Health and Human Services; 2008. http://www.health.gov/paguidelines/guidelines/default.aspx. Accessed September 19, 2017

US Department of Health and Human Services, US Department of Agriculture. *2015–2020 Dietary Guidelines for Americans*. 8th ed. Washington, DC: US Department of Health and Human Services; 2015. https://health.gov/dietaryguidelines/2015/resources/2015-2020_Dietary_Guidelines.pdf. Accessed September 19, 2017

RATIONALE

The *2015–2020 Dietary Guidelines for Americans and The Surgeon General's Call to Action to Support Breastfeeding* support patterns of healthy eating to promote a healthy weight and lifestyle that, in turn, prevent the onset of overweight and obesity in children (1,2). Incorporating each of the food groups by providing children with appropriate meals and snacks helps set the stage for a lifetime of healthy eating behaviors. Research reinforces

the following suggestions as being a practical approach to selecting foods high in essential nutrients and moderate in calories/energy:

- Meals and snacks planned based on the food groups in the Making Healthy Food Choices Table promote normal growth and development of children as well as reduce children's risk of overweight, obesity, and related chronic diseases later in life. Age-specific guidance for meals and snacks is outlined in the US Department of Agriculture Child and Adult Care Food Program (CACFP) guidelines (3).
- Early care and education settings provide the opportunity for children to learn about the food they eat, to develop and strengthen their fine and gross motor skills, and to engage in social interaction at mealtimes.
- "Energy" or sports beverages are typically high in added sugars and, therefore, not recommended for consumption. They contain many nonnutritive stimulants, such as caffeine, that have a history of harmful effects on a child's developing heart, brain, and nervous system (4).

COMMENTS

Early care and education settings should encourage mothers to breastfeed their infants. Scientific evidence documents and supports the nutritional and health contributions of human milk.[2] For more information on portion sizes and types of food, see the CACFP guidelines.[3]

RELATED STANDARDS

Meal and Snack Patterns
100% Fruit Juice
Feeding Plans and Dietary Modifications
Feeding Infants on Cue by a Consistent Caregiver/Teacher
Preparing, Feeding, and Storing Human Milk
Preparing, Feeding, and Storing Infant Formula
Feeding Cow's Milk
Meal and Snack Patterns for Toddlers and Preschoolers
Meal and Snack Patterns for School-Age Children
Nutrition Learning Experiences for Children
Nutrition Education for Parents/Guardians
Appendix: Getting Started with MyPlate
Appendix: Choose MyPlate: 10 Tips to a Great Plate

REFERENCES

1. US Department of Health and Human Services, US Department of Agriculture. *2015–2020 Dietary Guidelines for Americans. 8th ed. Washington, DC: US Department of Health and Human Services; 2015.* https://health.gov/dietaryguidelines/2015/resources/2015-2020_Dietary_Guidelines.pdf. Accessed September 19, 2017
2. US Department of Health and Human Services. *The Surgeon General's Call to Action to Support Breastfeeding.* Washington, DC: US Department of Health and Human Services, Office of the Surgeon General; 2011. https://www.cdc.gov/breastfeeding/promotion/calltoaction.htm. Updated April 12, 2017. Accessed September 19, 2017

Making Healthy Food Choices[a]		
Food Groups/ Ingredients	**USDA[b]**	**CFOC Guidelines for Young Children**
Fruits	**Whole Fruits** Includes fresh, frozen, canned (packed in water or 100% fruit juice), and dried varieties that include good sources of potassium (eg, bananas, dried plums) **Fruit Juice** 100% juice (ie, without added sugars)	• Eat a variety of whole fruits. • Whole fruit, mashed or pureed, for infants. • Do not serve juice to infants younger than 12 months. • No more than 4 oz of juice per day for 1- to 3-year-olds. • No more than 4–6 oz of juice per day for 4- to 6-year-olds. • No more than 8 oz of juice per day for 7- to 12-year-olds.
Vegetables	Includes fresh, frozen, canned, and dried varieties **Vegetable Subgroups** • Dark green • Red and orange Beans and peas (legumes) • Starchy vegetables • Other vegetables	• Include a variety of vegetables from the vegetable sub-groups. • Select low-sodium options when serving canned vegetables.
Grains	**Whole Grains** Contain the entire grain kernel (eg, whole wheat flour, bulgur, oatmeal, brown rice) **Refined Grains** Enriched grains that have been milled, processed, and stripped of vital nutrients	• Limit the amount of refined grains. • Make half the grains served whole grains or whole-grain products.
Protein Foods (Meat and Meat Alternatives)	Includes food from animal and plant sources (eg, seafood, lean meat, poultry, eggs, yogurt, cheese, soy products, nuts and seeds, cooked [mature] beans and peas)	• Fish, poultry, lean meat, eggs. • Unsalted nuts and seeds (if developmentally and age appropriate). • Legumes (beans and peas) may also be considered a protein source. • Limit processed meats and poultry. • Avoid fried fish and poultry.
Dairy	Fat-free or low-fat (1%) milk or soy milk	• Human milk and/or iron-fortified infant formula for infants 0–12 months of age. • Unflavored whole milk for children 1–2 years of age. • 2% (reduced-fat) milk for those children at risk for obesity or hypocholesteremia. • Unflavored low-fat (1%) or fat-free milk for children 2 years and older. • Nondairy milk substitutes that are nutritionally equivalent to milk. • Yogurt must not contain more than 23 g of sugar per ounce.

Abbreviations: CFOC, Caring for Our Children: National Health and Safety Performance Standards; USDA, US Department of Agriculture.

[a] All foods are assumed to be in nutrient-dense forms, lean or low-fat, and prepared without added fats, sugars, or salt. Solid fats and added sugars may be included up to the daily maximum limit identified in the 2015–2020 Dietary Guidelines for Americans.

[b] The USDA recommends finding a balance between food and physical activity.

3. US Department of Agriculture, Food and Nutrition Service. Child and Adult Care Food Program (CACFP). https://www.fns.usda.gov/cacfp/child-and-adult-care-food-program. Published March 29, 2017. Accessed September 19, 2017

4. Centers for Disease Control and Prevention. Healthy schools. The buzz on energy drinks. https://www.cdc.gov/healthyschools/nutrition/energy.htm. Updated March 22, 2016. Accessed September 19, 2017

NOTES

Content in the STANDARD was modified on 2/2012 and 11/16/2017.

Meal and Snack Patterns

The facility should ensure that the following meal and snack pattern occurs:

a. Children in care for 8 or fewer hours in 1 day should be offered at least 1 meal and 2 snacks or 2 meals and 1 snack (1).

b. A nutritious snack should be offered to all children in midmorning (if they are not offered a breakfast on-site that is provided within 3 hours of lunch) and in mid-afternoon.

c. Children should be offered food at intervals at least 2 hours apart but not more than 3 hours apart unless the child is asleep. Some very young infants may need to be fed at shorter intervals than every 2 hours to meet their nutritional needs, especially breastfed infants being fed expressed human milk. Lunch may need to be served to toddlers earlier than preschool-aged children because of their need for an earlier nap schedule. Children must be awake prior to being offered a meal/snack.

d. Children should be allowed time to eat their food and not be rushed during the meal or snack service. They should not be allowed to play during these times.

e. Caregivers/teachers should discuss breastfed infants' feeding patterns with their parents/guardians because the frequency of breastfeeding at home can vary. For example, some infants may still be feeding frequently at night, while others may do the bulk of their feeding during the day. Knowledge about infants' feeding patterns over 24 hours will help caregivers/teachers assess infants' feeding schedules during their time together.

RATIONALE

Children younger than 6 years need to be offered food every 2 to 3 hours. Appetite and interest in food varies from one meal or snack to the next. Appropriate timing of meals and snacks prevents children from snacking

throughout the day and ensures that children maintain healthy appetites during mealtimes (2,3). Snacks should be nutritious, as they often are a significant part of a child's daily intake. Children in care for longer than 8 hours need additional food because this period represents most of a young child's waking hours.

COMMENTS

Caloric needs vary greatly from one child to another. A child may require more food during growth spurts (4). Some states have regulations that indicate suggested times for meals and snacks. By regulation, under the US Department of Agriculture Child and Adult Care Food Program (CACFP), centers and family child care homes may be approved to claim up to 2 reimbursable meals (breakfast, lunch, or supper) and 1 snack, or 2 snacks and 1 meal, for each eligible participant, each day. Many after-school programs provide before-school care or full-day care when elementary school is out of session. Many of these programs offer breakfast and/or a morning snack. After-school care programs may claim reimbursement for serving each child one snack, each day. In some states after-school programs also have the option of providing supper. These are reimbursed by CACFP if they meet certain guidelines and time frames (5).

RELATED STANDARDS

Feeding Infants on Cue by a Consistent Caregiver/Teacher
Meal and Snack Patterns for Toddlers and Preschoolers
Meal and Snack Patterns for School-Age Children

REFERENCES

1. US Department of Agriculture, Food and Nutrition Service. *Independent Child Care Centers: A Child and Adult Care Food Program Handbook*. Washington, DC: US Department of Agriculture; 2014. https://www.fns.usda.gov/sites/default/files/cacfp/Independent%20Child%20Care%20Centers%20Handbook.pdf. Published May 2014. Accessed September 19, 2017

2. Shield JE, Mullen M. When should my kids snack? Academy of Nutrition and Dietetics Web site. http://www.eatright.org/resource/food/nutrition/dietary-guidelines-and-myplate/when-should-my-kids-snack. Published February 13, 2014. Accessed September 19, 2017

3. Kleinman RE, Greer FR, eds. *Pediatric Nutrition*. 7th ed. Elk Grove Village, IL: American Academy of Pediatrics; 2014

4. American Academy of Pediatrics Committee on Nutrition. Childhood nutrition. American Academy of Pediatrics HealthyChildren.org Web site. https://www.healthychildren.org/English/healthy-living/nutrition/Pages/Childhood-Nutrition.aspx. Updated March 3, 2016. Accessed September 19, 2017 US Department of Agriculture, Food and Nutrition Service. Child and Adult Care Food Program (CACFP). Why CACFP is important. https://www.fns.usda.gov/cacfp/why-cacfp-important. Published September 22, 2014. Accessed September 19, 2017

NOTES

Content in the STANDARD was modified on 11/9/2017.

Availability of Drinking Water

Clean, sanitary drinking water should be readily available, in indoor and outdoor areas, throughout the day (1). Water should not be a substitute for milk at meals or snacks where milk is a required food component unless recommended by the child's primary health care provider.

On hot days, infants receiving human milk in a bottle can be given additional human milk in a bottle but should not be given water, especially in the first 6 months after birth (1). Infants receiving formula and water can be given additional formula in a bottle. Toddlers and older children will need additional water as physical activity and/or hot temperatures cause their needs to increase. Children should learn to drink water from a cup or drinking fountain without mouthing the fixture. They should not be allowed to have water continuously in hand in a sippy cup or bottle. Permitting toddlers to suck continuously on a bottle or sippy cup filled with water, to soothe themselves, may cause nutritional or, in rare instances, electrolyte imbalances. When toothbrushing is not done after a feeding, children should be offered water to drink to rinse food from their teeth.

RATIONALE

When children are thirsty between meals and snacks, water is the best choice. Drinking water during the day can reduce extra caloric intake if the water replaces high-caloric beverages, such as fruit drinks/nectars and sodas, which are associated with overweight and obesity (2). Drinking water helps maintain a child's hydration and overall health. Water can also decrease the likelihood of early childhood caries if consumed throughout the day, especially between meals and snacks (3,4). Personal and environmental factors, such as age, weight, gender, physical activity level, outside air temperature, heat, and humidity, can affect individual water needs (5).

COMMENTS

Having clean, small pitchers of water and single-use paper cups available in classrooms and on playgrounds allows children to serve themselves water when they are thirsty. Drinking fountains should be kept clean and sanitary and maintained to provide adequate drainage.

RELATED STANDARDS

Playing Outdoors
Preparing, Feeding, and Storing Human Milk
Preparing, Feeding, and Storing Infant Formula

REFERENCES

1. Centers for Disease Control and Prevention. *Increasing Access to Drinking Water and Other Healthier Beverages in Early Care and Education Settings.* Atlanta, GA: US Department of Health and Human Services; 2014. https://www.cdc.gov/obesity/downloads/early-childhood-drinking-water-toolkit- final-508reduced.pdf. Accessed September 19, 2017
2. Muckelbauer R, Sarganas G, Grüneis A, Müller-Nordhorn J. Association between water consumption and body weight outcomes: a systematic review. *Am J Clin Nutr.* 2013;98(2):282–299
3. Kleinman RE, Greer FR, eds. *Pediatric Nutrition.* 7th ed. Elk Grove Village, IL: American Academy of Pediatrics; 2014
4. Casamassimo P, Holt K, eds. *Bright Futures: Oral Health Pocket Guide.* 3rd ed. Washington, DC: National Maternal and Child Oral Health Resource Center; 2016. https://www.mchoralhealth.org/PDFs/BFOHPocketGuide.pdf. Accessed September 19, 2017
5. Mullen M, Shield JE. Water: how much do kids need? Academy of Nutrition and Dietetics Web site. http://www.eatright.org/resource/fitness/sports-and- performance/hydrate-right/water-go-with-the-flow. Published May 2, 2017. Accessed September 19, 2017

NOTES

Content in the STANDARD was modified on 11/9/2017.

100% Fruit Juice

Fruit or vegetable juice may be served once per day during a scheduled meal or snack to children 12 months or older (1). All juices should be pasteurized and 100% juice without added sugars or sweeteners.

Age	Maximum Allowed[1]
0–12 mo	Do not offer juices to infants younger than 12 months.
1–3 y	Limit consumption to 4 oz/day (½ cup).
4–6 y	Limit consumption to 4–6 oz/day (½–¾ cup).
7–18 y	Limit consumption to 8 oz/day (1 cup).

100% juice should be offered in an age-appropriate cup instead of a bottle (2). These amounts include any juices consumed at home. Caregivers/teachers should ask parents/guardians if any juice is provided at home when deciding if and when to serve fruit juice to children in care. Whole fruit, mashed or pureed, is recommended for infants beginning at 4 months of age or as developmentally ready (3).

RATIONALE

While 100% fruit juice can be included in a healthy eating pattern, whole fruit is more nutritious and provides many nutrients, including dietary fiber, not found in juices (4).

Limiting overall juice consumption and encouraging children to drink water in-between meals will reduce acids produced by bacteria in the mouth that cause tooth decay. The frequency of exposure and liquids being pooled in the mouth are important in determining the cause of tooth decay in children (5). Beverages labeled as "fruit punch," "fruit nectar", or "fruit cocktail" contain less than 100% fruit juice and may be higher in overall sugar content. Routine consumption of fruit juices does not provide adequate amounts of vitamin E, iron, calcium, and dietary fiber—all essential in the growth and development of young children (6). Continuous consumption of fruit juice may be associated with decreased appetite during mealtimes, which may lead to inadequate nutrition, feeding issues, and increases in a child's body mass index—all of which are considered risk factors that may contribute to childhood obesity (7).

Serving pasteurized juice protects against the possible outbreak of foodborne illness because the process destroys any harmful bacteria that may have been present (8).

Drinks high in sugar and caffeine should be avoided because they can contribute to childhood obesity, tooth decay, and poor nutrition (9).

RELATED STANDARDS

Categories of Foods
Availability of Drinking Water
Introduction of Age-Appropriate Solid Foods to Infants

REFERENCES

1. Heyman MB, Abrams SA; American Academy of Pediatrics Section on Gastroenterology, Hepatology, and Nutrition and Committee on Nutrition. Fruit juice in infants, children, and adolescents: current recommendations. *Pediatrics*. 2017;139(6):e20170967
2. American Academy of Pediatrics. Fruit juice and your child's diet. American Academy of Pediatrics HealthyChildren.org Web site. https://www.healthychildren.org/English/healthy-living/nutrition/Pages/Fruit-Juice-and-Your-Childs-Diet.aspx. Updated May 22, 2017. Accessed September 19, 2017
3. American Academy of Pediatrics. Starting solid foods. American Academy of Pediatrics HealthyChildren.org Web site. https://www.healthychildren. org/English/ages-stages/baby/feeding-nutrition/Pages/Switching-To-Solid-Foods.aspx. Updated April 7, 2017. Accessed September 19, 2017
4. US Department of Health and Human Services, US Department of Agriculture. 2015–2020 Dietary Guidelines for Americans. 8th ed. Washington, DC: US Department of Health and Human Services; 2015. https://health.gov/dietaryguidelines/2015/resources/2015-2020_Dietary_ Guidelines.pdf. Accessed September 19, 2017
5. Casamassimo P, Holt K, eds. *Bright Futures: Oral Health Pocket Guide.* 3rd ed. Washington, DC: National Maternal and Child Oral Health Resource Center; 2016. https://www.mchoralhealth.org/PDFs/BFOHPocketGuide. pdf. Accessed September 19, 2017
6. Crowe-White K, O'Neil CE, Parrott JS, et al. Impact of 100% fruit juice consumption on diet and weight status of children: an evidence-based review. *Crit Rev Food Sci Nutr.* 2016;56(5):871–884
7. Shefferly A, Scharf RJ, DeBoer MD. Longitudinal evaluation of 100% fruit juice consumption on BMI status in 2–5-year-old children. *Pediatr Obes.* 2016;11(3):221–227
8. US Food and Drug Administration. Talking about juice safety: what you need to know. https://www.fda.gov/food/resourcesforyou/consumers/ucm110526.htm. Updated September 19, 2017. Accessed September 19, 2017
9. Centers for Disease Control and Prevention. Healthy schools. The buzz on energy drinks. https://www.cdc.gov/healthyschools/nutrition/energy.htm. Updated March 22, 2016. Accessed September 19, 2017.

NOTES

Content in the STANDARD was modified on 11/9/2017.

Written Menus and Introduction of New Foods

Facilities should develop, at least one month in advance, written menus that show all foods to be served during that month and should make the menus available to parents/guardians. The facility should date and retain these menus for 6 months, unless the state regulatory agency requires a longer retention time. The menus should be amended to reflect any and all changes in the food actually served. Any substitutions should be of equal nutrient value.

Caregivers/teachers should use or develop a take-home sheet for parents/guardians on which caregivers/teachers record the food consumed each day or, for breastfed infants, the number of times they are fed and other important notes. Caregivers/teachers should continue to consult with each infant's parent/guardian about foods they have introduced and are feeding to the infant. In this way, caregivers/teachers can follow a schedule of introducing new foods one at a time and more easily identify possible food allergies or intolerances. Caregivers/teachers should let parents/guardians know what and how much their infants eat each day.

To avoid problems of food sensitivity in infants younger than 12 months, caregivers/teachers should obtain from infants' parents/guardians a list of foods that have already been introduced (without any reaction) and serve those items when appropriate. As new foods are considered for serving, caregivers/teachers should share and discuss these foods with parents/guardians prior to their introduction.

RATIONALE

Planning menus in advance helps to ensure that food will be on hand. Posting menus in a prominent area and distributing them to parents/guardians helps to inform parents/guardians about proper nutrition Parents/guardians need to be informed about food served in the facility to know how to complement it with the food they serve at home. If a child has difficulty with any food served at the facility, parents/guardians can address this issue with appropriate staff members. Some regulatory agencies require menus as a part of the licensing and auditing process (1).

Consistency between home and the early care and education setting is essential during the period of rapid change when infants are learning to eat age-appropriate solid foods (1–3).

COMMENTS

Caregivers/teachers should be aware that new foods may need to be offered between 8 and 15 times before they may be accepted (2,4). Sample menus and menu planning templates are available from most state health departments and the US Department of Agriculture (5) and its Child and Adult Care Food Program (6).

Good communication between caregivers/teachers and parents/guardians is essential for successful feeding, in general, including when introducing age-appropriate solid foods (complementary foods). The decision to feed specific foods should be made in consultation with the parents/guardians. It is recommended that caregivers/teachers be given written instructions on the introduction and feeding of foods from the parents/guardians and the infants' primary health care providers.

RELATED STANDARDS

General Plan for Feeding Infants
Introduction of Age-Appropriate Solid Foods to Infants
Experience with Familiar and New Foods

REFERENCES

1. Benjamin SE, Copeland KA, Cradock A, et al. Menus in child care: a comparison of state regulations with national standards. *J Am Diet Assoc.* 2009;109(1):109–115
2. Coulthard H, Sealy A. Play with your food! Sensory play is associated with tasting of fruits and vegetables in preschool children. *Appetite.* 2017;113:84–90
3. Savage JS, Fisher JO, Birch LL. Parental influence on eating behavior: conception to adolescence. *J Law Med Ethics.* 2007;35(1):22–34
4. US Department of Agriculture. Menu planning tools for child care providers. https://healthymeals.fns.usda.gov/menu-planning/menu-planning-tools/menu-planning-tools-child-care-providers. Accessed September 20, 2017
5. US Department of Agriculture, Food and Nutrition Service. Child and Adult Care Food Program (CACFP). https://www.fns.usda.gov/cacfp/child-and-adult-care-food-program. Published March 29, 2017. Accessed September 20, 2017
6. American Academy of Pediatrics Committee on Nutrition. Childhood nutrition. American Academy of Pediatrics HealthyChildren.org Web site. https://www.healthychildren.org/English/healthy-living/nutrition/Pages/Childhood-Nutrition.aspx. Updated March 3, 2016. Accessed September 20, 2017

NOTES

Content in the STANDARD was modified on 11/9/2017.

Care for Children with Food Allergies

When children with food allergies attend an early care and education facility, here is what should occur.

a. Each child with a food allergy should have a care plan prepared for the facility by the child's primary health care provider, to include

   1. A written list of the food(s) to which the child is allergic and instructions for steps that need to be taken to avoid that food.
   2. A detailed treatment plan to be implemented in the event of an allergic reaction, including the names, doses, and methods of administration of any medications that the child should receive in the event of a reaction. The plan should include specific symptoms that would indicate the need to administer one or more medications.

b. Based on the child's care plan, the child's caregivers/teachers should receive training, demonstrate competence in, and implement measures for

   1. Preventing exposure to the specific food(s) to which the child is allergic
   2. Recognizing the symptoms of an allergic reaction
   3. Treating allergic reactions

c. Parents/guardians and staff should arrange for the facility to have the necessary medications, proper storage of such medications, and the equipment and training to manage the child's food allergy while the child is at the early care and education facility.

d. Caregivers/teachers should promptly and properly administer prescribed medications in the event of an allergic reaction according to the instructions in the care plan.

e. The facility should notify parents/guardians immediately of any suspected allergic reactions, the ingestion of the problem food, or contact with the problem food, even if a reaction did not occur.

f. The facility should recommend to the family that the child's primary health care provider be notified if the child has required treatment by the facility for a food allergic reaction.

g. The facility should contact the emergency medical services (EMS) system immediately if the child has any serious allergic reaction and/or whenever epinephrine (eg, EpiPen, EpiPen Jr) has been administered, even if the child appears to have recovered from the allergic reaction.

h. Parents/guardians of all children in the child's class should be advised to avoid any known allergens in class treats or special foods brought into the early care and education setting.

i. Individual child's food allergies should be posted prominently in the classroom where staff can view them and/or wherever food is served.

j. The written child care plan, a mobile phone, and a list of the proper medications for appropriate treatment if the child develops an acute allergic reaction should be routinely carried on field trips or transport out of the early care and education setting.

For all children with a history of anaphylaxis (severe allergic reaction), or for those with peanut and/or tree nut allergy (whether or not they have had anaphylaxis), epinephrine should be readily available. This will usually be provided as a premeasured dose in an auto-injector, such as EpiPen or EpiPen Jr. Specific indications for administration of epinephrine should be provided in the detailed care plan. Within the context of state laws, appropriate personnel should be prepared to administer epinephrine when needed.

Food sharing between children must be prevented by careful supervision and repeated instruction to children about this issue. Exposure may also occur through contact between children or by contact with contaminated surfaces, such as a table on which the food allergen remains after eating. Some children may have an allergic reaction just from being in proximity to the offending food, without actually ingesting it. Such contact should be minimized by washing children's hands and faces and all surfaces that were in contact with food. In addition, reactions may occur when a food is used as part of an art or craft project, such as the use of peanut butter to make a bird feeder or wheat to make modeling compound.

RATIONALE

Food allergy is common, occurring in between 2% and 8% of infants and children (1). Allergic reactions to food can range from mild skin or gastrointestinal symptoms to severe, life-threatening reactions with respiratory and/or cardiovascular compromise. Hospitalizations from food allergy are being reported in increasing numbers, especially among children with asthma who have one or more food sensitivities (2). A major factor in death from anaphylaxis has been a delay in the administration of lifesaving emergency medication, particularly epinephrine (3). Intensive efforts to avoid exposure to the offending food(s) are, therefore, warranted. The maintenance of detailed care plans and the ability to implement such plans for the treatment of reactions are essential for all children with food allergies (4).

COMMENTS

Successful food avoidance requires a cooperative effort that must include the parents/guardians, child, child's primary health care provider, and early care and education staff. In some cases, especially for a child with multiple food allergies, parents/guardians may need to take responsibility for providing all the child's food. In other cases, early care and education staff may be able to provide safe foods as long as they have been fully educated about effective food avoidance.

Effective food avoidance has several facets. Foods can be listed on an ingredient list under a variety of names; for example, milk could be listed as casein, caseinate, whey, and/or lactoglobulin.

Some children with a food allergy will have mild reactions and will only need to avoid the problem food(s). Others will need to have antihistamine or epinephrine available to be used in the event of a reaction.

For more information on food allergies, contact Food Allergy Research & Education (FARE) at www.foodallergy.org. Some early care and education/school settings require that all foods brought into the classroom are store-bought and in their original packaging so that a list of ingredients is included, to prevent exposure to allergens. However, packaged foods may mistakenly include allergen-type ingredients. Alerts and ingredient recalls can be found on the FARE Web site (5).

RELATED STANDARDS
Assessment and Planning of Nutrition for Individual Children
Feeding Plans and Dietary Modifications

REFERENCES

1. Bugden EA, Martinez AK, Greene BZ, Eig K. *Safe at School and Ready to Learn: A Comprehensive Policy Guide for Protecting Students with Life-threatening Food Allergies.* 2nd ed. Alexandria, VA: National School Boards Association; 2012. http://www.nsba.org/sites/default/files/reports/Safe-at-School-and-Ready-to-Learn.pdf. Accessed September 20, 2017
2. Caffarelli C, Garrubba M, Greco C, Mastrorilli C, Povesi Dascola C. Asthma and food allergy in children: is there a connection or interaction? *Front Pediatr.* 2016;4:34
3. Tsuang A, Demain H, Patrick K, Pistiner M, Wang J. Epinephrine use and training in schools for food-induced anaphylaxis among non-nursing staff. *J Allergy Clin Immunol Pract.* 2017;5(5):1418–1420.e3
4. Wang J, Sicherer SH; American Academy of Pediatrics Section on Allergy and Immunology. Guidance on completing a written allergy and anaphylaxis emergency plan. *Pediatrics.* 2017;139(3):e20164005
5. Food Allergy Research & Education. Allergy alerts. https://www.foodallergy.org/alerts. Accessed September 20, 2017

ADDITIONAL RESOURCES

Centers for Disease Control and Prevention. Healthy schools. Food allergies in schools. https://www.cdc.gov/healthyschools/foodallergies/index.htm. Reviewed May 9, 2017. Accessed September 20, 2017

Centers for Disease Control and Prevention. *Voluntary Guidelines for Managing Food Allergies in Schools and Early Care and Education Programs.* Washington, DC: US Department of Health and Human Services; 2013. https://www.cdc.gov/healthyschools/foodallergies/pdf/13_243135_A_Food_Allergy_Web_508.pdf. Accessed September 20, 2017

NOTES

Content in the STANDARD was modified on 11/9/2017.

Ingestion of Substances that Do Not Provide Nutrition

All children should be monitored to prevent them from eating substances that do not provide nutrition (often referred to as pica) (1,2). The parents/guardians of children who repeatedly place nonnutritive substances in their mouths should be notified and informed of the importance of having their children visit their primary health care provider or a local health department. In collaboration with the child's parent/guardian, an assessment of the child's eating behavior and dietary intake, along with any other health issues, should occur to begin an intervention strategy.

RATIONALE

The occasional ingestion of nonnutritive substances can be a part of everyday living and is not necessarily a concern. For example, ingestion of nonnutritive substances can occur from mouthing, placing dirty hands in the mouth, or eating dropped food. However, because of this normal behavior it is that much more important to minimize harmful residues in the facility to reduce children's exposure. Pica involves the recurrent ingestion of substances that do not provide nutrition. Pica is most prevalent among children between the ages of 1 and 3 years (3). Among children with intellectual developmental disability and concurrent mental illness, the incidence exceeds 25% (3).

Children who have iron deficiency anemia regularly ingest nonnutritive substances. Dietary intake plays an important role because certain nutrients, such as those ingested with a diet high in fat or lecithin, increase the absorption of lead, which can result in toxicity (3). Lead, when present in the gastrointestinal tract, is absorbed in place of calcium.

Children will absorb more lead than an adult. Whereas an adult absorbs approximately 10% of ingested lead, a toddler absorbs approximately 30% to 50% of ingested lead. Children who ingest paint chips or contaminated soil can develop lead toxicity, which can lead to developmental delays and neurodevelopmental disability. Currently, there is consensus that repeated ingestion of some nonfood items results in an increased lead burden of the body (3,4). Early detection and intervention in nonfood ingestion can prevent nutritional deficiencies and growth/developmental disabilities. Eating soil or drinking contaminated water could result in an infection with a parasite.

COMMENTS

Common sources of lead include lead-based paint (in buildings constructed before 1978 or constructed on properties that were formerly the site of buildings constructed before 1978); contaminated drinking water (from public water systems, supply pipes, or plumbing fixtures); contaminated soil (from old exterior paint); the storage of acidic foods in open cans or ceramic containers/pottery with a lead glaze; certain types of art supplies; some imported toys and inexpensive play jewelry; and polyvinyl chloride (PVC) vinyl products (eg, beach balls, soft PVC-containing dolls, rubber ducks, chew toys, nap mats). These sources and others should be addressed concurrently with a nutritionally adequate diet as a prevention strategy. It is important to reduce exposure to possible lead sources, promote a healthy and balanced diet, and encourage blood lead level (BLL) testing of children. If a child's BLL is 5 mcg/dL or greater, it is important to identify and remove the child's source of lead exposure.

REFERENCES

1. Centers for Disease Control and Prevention. Gateway to health communication & social marketing practice. Pica behavior and contaminated soil. https://www.cdc.gov/healthcommunication/toolstemplates/entertainmented/tips/pica.html. Updated September 15, 2017. Accessed September 20, 2017
2. Miao D, Young SL, Golden CD. A meta-analysis of pica and micronutrient status. *Am J Hum Biol.* 2015;27(1):84–93
3. McNaughten B, Bourke T, Thompson A. Fifteen-minute consultation: the child with pica. *Arch Dis Child Educ Pract Ed.* May 2017;edpract-2016-312121
4. Moya J, Bearer CF, Etzel RA. Children's behavior and physiology and how it affects exposure to environmental contaminants. *Pediatrics.* 2004;113(4 Suppl 3):996–1006

NOTES

Content in this STANDARD was modified on August 23, 2016 and November 10, 2017.

Vegetarian/Vegan Diets

Infants and children, including school-aged children from families practicing a vegetarian diet, can be accommodated in an early care and education environment when there is:

a. Written documentation from parents/guardians with a detailed and accurate dietary history of food choices— foods eaten, levels of limitations/restrictions to foods, and frequency of foods offered;

b. A current health record of the child available to the caregivers/teachers, including information about height and rate of weight gain, or consistent poor appetite (warning signs of growth deficiencies);

c. Sharing of updated information on the child's health with the parents/guardians and the early care and education staff by the child care health consultant and the nutritionist/registered dietitian; and

d. Sharing sound health and nutrition information that is culturally-relevant to the family to ensure that the child receives adequate calories and essential nutrients.

RATIONALE

Infants and young children are at highest risk for nutritional deficiencies for energy levels and essential nutrients, including protein, calcium, iron, zinc, vitamins B and B, and vitamin D (1–3). The younger the child, the more critical it is to know about family food 6 12 choices, limitations, and restrictions because the child is dependent on family food (2).

Also, it is important that a child's diet consist of a variety of nourishing food to support the critical period of rapid growth in the early years after birth. All children who are vegetarian/vegan should receive multivitamins, especially vitamin D (400 IU of vitamin D is recommended from

6 months of age to adulthood unless there is certainty of having the daily allowance met by foods); infants younger than 6 months who are exclusively or partially breastfed and who receive less than 16 oz of formula per day should receive 400 IU of vitamin D (4). If the facility participates in the US Department of Agriculture Child and Adult Care Food Program, guidance for meals and snack patterns must be followed for any child consuming a vegetarian or vegan diet (5).

COMMENTS

For older children who have more choice about what they eat and drink, effort should be made to provide accurate nutrition information so they make the wisest food choices for themselves. Both the early care and education program/school and the caregiver/teacher have an opportunity to inform, teach, and promote sound eating practices, along with the consequences when poor food choices are made (1). Sensitivity to cultural factors, including beliefs and practices of a child's family, should be maintained.

Changing lifestyles and convictions and beliefs about food and religion, including what is eaten and what foods are restricted or never consumed, have some families with infants and children practicing several levels of vegetarian diets. Some parents/guardians indicate they are vegetarians, semi-vegetarian, or strict vegetarians because they do not or seldom eat meat. Others label themselves lacto-ovo vegetarians, eating or drinking foods such as eggs and dairy products. Still others describe themselves as vegans who restrict themselves to ingesting only plant-based foods, avoiding all and any animal products.

RELATED STANDARDS

Routine Health Supervision and Growth Monitoring
Assessment and Planning of Nutrition for Individual Children
Use of Soy-Based Formula and Soy Milk
Use of Nutritionist/Registered Dietitian

REFERENCES

1. Kleinman RE, Greer FR, eds. *Pediatric Nutrition.* 7th ed. Elk Grove Village, IL: American Academy of Pediatrics; 2014
2. Hayes D. *Feeding vegetarian and vegan infants and toddlers.* Academy of Nutrition and Dietetics Web site. http://www.eatright.org/resource/food/nutrition/vegetarian-and-special-diets/feeding-vegetarian-and-vegan-infants-and-toddlers. Published May 4, 2015. Accessed September 20, 2017
3. Mangels R, Driggers J. The youngest vegetarians. Vegetarian infants and toddlers. *Infant Child Adolesc Nutr.* 2012;4(1):8–20

4. Hollis BW, Wagner CL, Howard CR, et al. Maternal versus infant vitamin D supplementation during lactation: a randomized controlled trial. *Pediatrics*. 2015;136(4):625–634

5. US Department of Agriculture, Food and Nutrition Service. *Independent Child Care Centers: A Child and Adult Care Food Program Handbook*. Washington, DC: US Department of Agriculture; 2014. https://www.fns. usda.gov/sites/default/files/cacfp/Independent%20 Child%20Care%20 Centers%20Handbook.pdf. Accessed September 20, 2017

ADDITIONAL RESOURCES

US Department of Agriculture. 10 tips: healthy eating for vegetarians. ChooseMyPlate.gov Web site. https://www.choosemyplate.gov/ ten-tips-healthy-eating-for-vegetarians. Updated July 25, 2017. Accessed September 20, 2017

US Department of Agriculture, US Department of Health and Human Services. Meat and meat alternates: build a healthy plate with protein. In: *Nutrition and Wellness Tips for Young Children: Provider Handbook for the Child and Adult Care Food Program*. Alexandria, VA: US Department of Agriculture; 2012. https://www.fns.usda.gov/sites/default/files/protein. pdf. Accessed September 20, 2017

NOTES

Content in this STANDARD was modified on November 10, 2017.

Requirements for Infants

General Plan for Feeding Infants

The facility should keep records detailing whether an infant is breastfed or formula fed, along with the type of formula being served. An infant feeding record of human (breast) milk and/or all formula given to the infant should be completed daily. Infant meals and snacks should follow the meal and snack patterns of the Child and Adult Care Food Program. Food should be appropriate for the infant's individual nutrition requirements and developmental stage as determined by written instructions obtained from the child's parent/guardian or primary health care provider.

The facility should encourage breastfeeding by providing accommodations and continuous support to the breastfeeding mother. Facilities should have a designated place set aside for breastfeeding mothers who want to visit the classroom during the workday to breastfeed, as well as a private area (not a bathroom) with an outlet for mothers to pump their breast milk (1,2). The private area also should have access to water or hand hygiene. A place that parents/guardians feel they are welcome to breastfeed, pump, or bottle-feed can create a positive and supportive environment for the family.

Infants may need a variety of special formulas, such as soy-based formula or elemental formulas, that are easier to digest and less allergenic. Elemental or special hypoallergenic formulas should be specified in the infant's care plan. Age-appropriate solid foods other than human milk or infant formula (ie, *complementary* foods) should be introduced no sooner than 6 months of age or as indicated by the individual child's nutritional and developmental needs. Please refer to Introduction of Age-Appropriate Solid Foods and Feeding Age-Appropriate Solid Foods to Infants for more information.

RATIONALE

Human milk, as an exclusive food, is best suited to meet the entire nutritional needs of an infant from birth until 6 months of age, with the exception of recommended vitamin D supplementation. In addition to nutrition, breastfeeding supports optimal health and development. Human milk is also the best source of milk for infants for at least the first 12 months of age and, thereafter, for as long as mutually desired by mother and child. Breastfeeding protects infants from many acute and chronic diseases and has advantages for the mother, as well (3).

Research overwhelmingly shows that exclusive breastfeeding for 6 months, and continued breastfeeding for at least a year or longer, dramatically improves health outcomes for children and their mothers. Healthy People 2020 outlines several objectives, including increasing the proportion of mothers who breastfeed their infants and increasing the duration of breastfeeding and exclusive breastfeeding (4).

Incidences of common childhood illnesses, such as diarrhea, respiratory disease, bacterial meningitis, botulism, urinary tract infections, sudden infant death syndrome, insulin-dependent diabetes, ulcerative colitis, and ear infections, and overall risk for childhood obesity are significantly decreased in breastfed children (5,6). Similarly, breastfeeding, when paired with other healthy parenting behaviors, has been directly related to increased cognitive development in infants (7). Breastfeeding also has added benefits to the mother: it decreases risk of diabetes, breast and ovarian cancers, and heart disease (8).

Mothers who want to supplement their breast milk with formula may do so, as the infant will continue to receive breastfeeding benefits (4,5,7). Iron-fortified infant formula is an acceptable alternative to human milk as a food for infant feeding even though it lacks any anti-infective or immunological components. Regardless of feeding preference, an adequately nourished infant is more likely to achieve healthy physical and mental development, which will have long-term positive effects on health (9).

COMMENTS

The ways to help a mother breastfeed successfully in the early care and education facility are (2,6,8):

a. If she wishes to breastfeed her infant or child when she comes to the facility, offer or provide her a
   1. Quiet, comfortable, and private place to breastfeed (This helps her milk to let down.)
   2. Place to wash her and her infant's hands before and after breastfeeding
   3. Pillow to support her infant on her lap while nursing
   4. Nursing stool or step stool for her feet so she doesn't have to strain her back while nursing
   5. Glass of water or other liquid to help her stay hydrated
b. Encourage her to get the infant used to being fed her expressed human milk by another person before the infant starts in early care and education, while continuing to breastfeed directly herself.
c. Discuss with her the infant's usual feeding pattern and the benefits of feeding the infant based on the infant's hunger and satiety cues rather than on a schedule; ask her if she wishes to time the infant's last feeding so that the infant is hungry and ready to breastfeed when she arrives; and ask her to leave her availability schedule with the early care and education program as well as to call if she is planning to miss a feeding or is going to be late.
d. Encourage her to provide a backup supply of frozen or refrigerated expressed human milk; properly label the infant's full name, date, and time on the bottle or other clean storage container in case the infant needs to eat more often than usual or the mother's visit is delayed.
e. Share with her information about other places or people in the community who can answer her questions and concerns about breastfeeding, such as local lactation consultants.
   1. Provide culturally appropriate breastfeeding materials, including community resources for parents/guardians that include appropriate language and pictures of multicultural families to assist families in identifying with them.
f. Ensure that all staff receive training in breastfeeding support and promotion.
g. Ensure that all staff are trained in the proper handling, storing, and feeding of each milk product, including human milk or infant formula.

ADDITIONAL RESOURCES

Breastfeeding, US Department of Health and Human Services Office on Women's Health (https://www.womenshealth.gov/printables-and-shareables/health-topic/breastfeeding)

Feeding Infants: A Guide for Use in the Child Nutrition Programs, US Department of Agriculture (USDA) Food and Nutrition Service (https://www. fns.usda.gov/tn/feeding-infants-guide-use-child-nutrition-programs)

Infant Meal Pattern, USDA (https://fns-prod.azureedge.net/sites/default/files/cacfp/CACFP_infantmealpattern.pdf)

Strategy 6, Support for Breastfeeding in Early Care and Education, Centers for Disease Control and Prevention (https://www.cdc.gov/breastfeeding/pdf/strategy6-support-breastfeeding-early-care.pdf)

Updated Child and Adult Care Food Program Meal Patterns: Infant Meals, USDA (https://fns-prod.azureedge.net/sites/default/files/cacfp/CACFP_InfantMealPattern_FactSheet_V2.pdf)

RELATED STANDARDS

Written Menus and Introduction of New Foods
Preparing, Feeding, and Storing Human Milk
Preparing, Feeding, and Storing Infant Formula
Introduction of Age-Appropriate Solid Foods to Infants
Feeding Age-Appropriate Solid Foods to Infants
Appendix: Our Child Care Center Supports Breastfeeding

REFERENCES

1. Centers for Disease Control and Prevention. Strategies to Prevent Obesity and Other Chronic Diseases: The CDC Guide to Strategies to Support Breastfeeding Mothers and Babies. Atlanta, GA: US Department of Health and Human Services; 2013. http://www.cdc.gov/breastfeeding/pdf/BF-Guide-508.pdf. Accessed January 11, 2018
2. Special Supplemental Nutrition Program for Women, Infants, and Children (WIC); US Department of Agriculture Food and Nutrition Service. Breastfeeding Policy and Guidance. https://www.fns.usda.gov/sites/default/files/wic/WIC-Breastfeeding-Policy-and-Guidance.pdf. Published July 2016. Accessed January 11, 2018
3. Darmawikarta D, Chen Y, Lebovic G, Birken CS, Parkin PC, Maguire JL. Total duration of breastfeeding, vitamin D supplementation, and serum levels of 25-hydroxyvitamin D. *Am J Public Health.* 2016;106(4):714–719
4. Healthy People 2020. Maternal, infant, and child health. HealthyPeople.gov Web site. https://www.healthypeople.gov/2020/topics-objectives/topic/maternal-infant-and-child-health/objectives. Accessed January 11, 2018
5. Furman L. Breastfeeding: what do we know, and where do we go from here? *Pediatrics.* 2017;139(4):e20170150
6. American Academy of Pediatrics Section on Breastfeeding. Breastfeeding and the use of human milk. *Pediatrics.* 2012;129(3):e827–e841
7. Gibbs BG, Forste R. Breastfeeding, parenting, and early cognitive development. *J Pediatr.* 2014;164(3):487–493
8. Binns C, Lee M, Low WY. The long-term public health benefits of breastfeeding. *Asia Pac J Public Health.* 2016;28(1):7–14
9. Danawi H, Estrada L, Hasbini T, Wilson DR. Health inequalities and breastfeeding in the United States of America. *Int J Childbirth Educ.* 2016;31(1)

NOTES

Content in the STANDARD was modified on 05/30/2018.

Feeding Infants on Cue by a Consistent Caregiver/Teacher

Caregivers/teachers should feed infants on cue unless the parent/guardian and the child's primary health care provider give written instructions stating otherwise (1). Caregivers/teachers should be gentle, patient, sensitive, and reassuring when responding appropriately to the infant's feeding cues (2). Responsive feeding is most successful when caregivers/teachers learn how infants externally communicate hunger and fullness. Crying alone is not a cue for hunger unless accompanied by other cues, such as opening the mouth, making sucking sounds, rooting, fast breathing, clenched fingers/fists, and flexed arms/legs (1,2). Whenever possible, the same caregiver/teacher should feed a specific infant for most of that infant's feedings (3). Caregivers/teachers should not feed infants beyond satiety; just as hunger cues are important in initiating feedings, observing satiety cues can limit overfeeding. An infant will communicate fullness by shaking the head or turning away from food (1,4,5).

A pacifier should not be offered to an infant prior to being fed.

RATIONALE

Responsive feeding meets the infant's nutritional and emotional needs and provides an immediate response to the infant, which helps ensure trust and feelings of security (6). A caregiver/teacher is more likely to understand how a particular infant communicates hunger/satiety when consistent, reliable feedings and interactions are done regularly over time. Early relationships between an infant and caregivers/teachers involving feeding set the stage for an infant to develop eating patterns for life (1–5). Responsive feeding may help prevent childhood obesity (5–7).

RELATED STANDARDS

General Plan for Feeding Infants
Techniques for Bottle Feeding

REFERENCES

1. Blaine RE, Davison KK, Hesketh K, Taveras EM, Gillman MW, Benjamin Neelon SE. Child care provider adherence to infant and toddler feeding recommendations: findings from the Baby Nutrition and Physical Activity Self-Assessment for Child Care (Baby NAP SACC) Study. *Child Obes*. 2015;11(3):304–313

2. Pérez-Escamilla R, Segura-Pérez S, Lott M, on behalf of the Robert Wood Johnson Foundation HER Expert Panel on Best Practices for Promoting Healthy Nutrition, Feeding Patterns, and Weight Status for Infants and Toddlers From Birth to 24 Months. Feeding Guidelines for Infants and Young Toddlers: A Responsive Parenting Approach. Guidelines for Health Professionals. Durham, NC: Healthy Eating Research; 2017. http://healthyeatingresearch.org/wp-content/uploads/2017/02/her_feeding_guidelines_brief_021416.pdf. Published February 2017. Accessed November 14, 2017

3. Zero to Three. How to care for infants and toddlers in groups. 4. Continuity of care. https://www.zerotothree.org/resources/77-how-to-care-for-infants- and-toddlers-in-groups#chapter-38. Published February 8, 2010. Accessed November 14, 2017

4. US Department of Agriculture, Special Supplemental Nutrition Program for Women, Infants, and Children. Infant hunger and satiety cues. https://wicworks.fns.usda.gov/wicworks/WIC_Learning_Online/support/job_aids/cues.pdf. Updated October 2016. Accessed November 14, 2017

5. Buvinger E, Rosenblum K, Miller AL, Kaciroti NA, Lumeng JC. Observed infant food cue responsivity: associations with maternal report of infant eating behavior, breastfeeding, and infant weight-gain. *Appetite*. 2017;112:219–226

6. Early Head Start National Resource Center. Observation: The Heart of Individualizing Responsive Care. Washington, DC: Early Head Start National Resource Center; 2013. https://eclkc.ohs.acf.hhs.gov/sites/default/files/pdf/ehs-ta-paper-15-observation.pdf. Accessed November 14, 2017

7. Redsell SA, Edmonds B, Swift JA, et al. Systematic review of randomised controlled trials of interventions that aim to reduce the risk, either directly or indirectly, of overweight and obesity in infancy and early childhood. *Matern Child Nutr*. 2016;12(1):24–38

NOTES

Content in the STANDARD was modified on 05/30/2018.

Preparing, Feeding, and Storing Human Milk

Expressed human milk should be placed in a clean and sanitary bottle with a nipple that fits tightly or into an equivalent clean and sanitary sealed container to prevent spilling during transport to home or to the facility. Only cleaned and sanitized bottles, or their equivalent, and nipples should be used in feeding. The bottle or container should be properly labeled with the infant's full name and the date and time the milk was expressed. The bottle or container should immediately be stored in the refrigerator on arrival.

The mother's own expressed milk should only be used for her own infant. Likewise, infant formula should not be used for a breastfed infant without the mother's written permission.

Avoid bottles made of plastics containing bisphenol A (BPA) or phthalates, sometimes labeled with #3, #6, or #7 (1). Use glass bottles with a silicone sleeve (a silicone bottle jacket to prevent breakage) or those made with safer plastics such as polypropylene or polyethylene (labeled BPA-free) or plastics with a recycling code of #1, #2, #4, or #5.

Non-frozen human milk should be transported and stored in the containers to be used to feed the infant, identified with a label which will not come off in water or handling, bearing the date of collection and child's full name. The filled, labeled containers of human milk should be kept refrigerated. Human milk containers with significant amount of contents remaining (greater than one ounce) may be returned to the mother at the end of the day as long as the child has not fed directly from the bottle.

Frozen human milk may be transported and stored in single use plastic bags and placed in a freezer (not a compartment within a refrigerator but either a freezer with a separate door or a standalone freezer). Human milk should be defrosted in the refrigerator if frozen, and then heated briefly in bottle warmers or under warm running water so that the temperature does not exceed 98.6°F. If there is insufficient time to defrost the milk in the refrigerator before warming it, then it may be defrosted in a container of running cool tap water, very gently swirling the bottle periodically to evenly distribute the temperature

in the milk. Some infants will not take their mother's milk unless it is warmed to body temperature, around 98.6°F. The caregiver/teacher should check for the infant's full name and the date on the bottle so that the oldest milk is used first. After warming, bottles should be mixed gently (not shaken) and the temperature of the milk tested before feeding.

Expressed human milk that presents a threat to an infant, such as human milk that is in an unsanitary bottle, is curdled, smells rotten, and/or has not been stored following the storage guidelines of the Academy of Breastfeeding Medicine as shown later in this standard, should be returned to the mother.

Some children around six months to a year of age may be developmentally ready to feed themselves and may want to drink from a cup. The transition from bottle to cup can come at a time when a child's fine motor skills allow use of a cup. The caregiver/teacher should use a clean small cup without cracks or chips and should help the child to lift and tilt the cup to avoid spillage and leftover fluid. The caregiver/teacher and mother should work together on cup feeding of human milk to ensure the child is receiving adequate nourishment and to avoid having a large amount of human milk remaining at the end of feeding. Two to three ounces of human milk can be

Guidelines for Storage of Human Milk			
Location	**Temperature**	**Duration**	**Comments**
Countertop, table	Room temperature (up to 77°F or 25°C)	6–8 hours	Containers should be covered and kept as cool as possible; covering the container with a cool towel may keep milk cooler.
Insulated cooler bag	5°F–39°F or −15°C–4°C	24 hours	Keep ice packs in contact with milk containers at all times, limit opening cooler bag.
Refrigerator	39°F or 4°C	5 days	Store milk in the back of the main body of the refrigerator.
Freezer compartment of a refrigerator	5°F or −15°C	2 weeks	Store milk toward the back of the freezer, where temperature is most constant. Milk stored for longer durations in the ranges listed is safe, but some of the lipids in the milk undergo degradation resulting in lower quality.
Freezer compartment of refrigerator with separate doors	0°F or −18°C	3–6 months	
Chest or upright deep freezer	−4°F or −20°C	6–12 months	

Source: Academy of Breastfeeding Medicine Protocol Committee. 2010. Clinical protocol #8: Human milk storage information for home use for healthy full term infants, revised. Breastfeeding Med 5:127-30. http://www.bfmed.org/Media/Files/Protocols/Protocol%208%20-%20English%20revised%20 2010.pdf.

From the Centers for Disease Control and Prevention Website: Proper handling and storage of human milk – Storage duration of fresh human milk for use with healthy full term infants. http://www.cdc.gov/breastfeeding/recommendations/handling_breastmilk.htm.

placed in a clean cup and additional milk can be offered as needed. Small amounts of human milk (about an ounce) can be discarded.

Human milk can be stored using the guidelines from the Academy of Breastfeeding Medicine on the previous page.

RATIONALE

Labels for containers of human milk should be resistant to loss of the name and date/time when washing and handling. This is especially important when the frozen bottle is thawed in running tap water. There may be several bottles from different mothers being thawed and warmed at the same time in the same place.

By following this standard, the staff is able, when necessary, to prepare human milk and feed an infant safely, thereby reducing the risk of inaccuracy or feeding the infant unsanitary or incorrect human milk (2,3). Written guidance for both staff and parents/guardians should be available to determine when milk provided by parents/guardians will not be served. Human milk cannot be served if it does not meet the requirements for sanitary and safe milk.

Although human milk is a body fluid, it is not necessary to wear gloves when feeding or handling human milk. Unless there is visible blood in the milk, the risk of exposure to infectious organisms either during feeding or from milk that the infant regurgitates is not significant.

Returning unused human milk to the mother informs her of the quantity taken while in the early care and education program.

Excessive shaking of human milk may damage some of the cellular components that are valuable to the infant. It is difficult to maintain 0°F consistently in a freezer compartment of a refrigerator or freezer, so caregivers/teachers should carefully monitor, with daily log sheets, temperature of freezers used to store human milk using an appropriate working thermometer. Human milk contains components that are damaged by excessive heating during or after thawing from the frozen state (4). Currently, there is nothing in the research literature that states that feedings must be warmed at all prior to feeding. Frozen milk should never be thawed in a microwave oven as 1) uneven hot spots in the milk may cause burns in the infant and 2) excessive heat may destroy beneficial components of the milk.

By following safe preparation and storage techniques, nursing mothers and caregivers/teachers of breastfed infants and children can maintain the high quality of expressed human milk and the health of the infant (5,6).

RELATED STANDARDS

General Plan for Feeding Infants
Feeding Human Milk to Another Mother's Child
Feeding Cow's Milk
Techniques for Bottle Feeding
Warming Bottles and Infant Foods

REFERENCES

1. Harley, K.G., Gunier, R.B., Kogut, K., Johnson, C., et al. 2013. Prenatal and early childhood bisphenol a concentrations and behavior in school-aged children. *Environ Res.* 126: 43–50.
2. United States Cooperative Expansion System. 2015. *Guidelines for child care providers to prepare and feed bottles to infants. 2015.* http://articles. extension.org/pages/25404/guidelines-for-child-care-providers-to-prepare-and-feed-bottles-to-infants.
3. Centers for Disease Control and Prevention. 2016. Proper handling and storage of human milk. Atlanta, GA. https://www.cdc.gov/breastfeeding/recommendations/handling_breastmilk.htm.
4. La Leche League International. (2014). Storage guidelines: LLLI guidelines for storing breastmilk. http://www.llli.org/faq/milkstorage.html.
5. Boué, G., Cummins, E., Guillou, S., Antignac, J., Bizec, B., & Membré, J. 2016. Public health risks and benefits associated with breast milk and infant formula consumption. *Critical Reviews in Food Science and Nutrition.* Feb 6:1–20.
6. Binns, C. 2016. The long-term public health benefits of breastfeeding. *Asia-Pacific Journal of Public Health.* 28(1):7.

NOTES

Content in the STANDARD was modified on 8/23/2016.

Feeding Human Milk to Another Mother's Child

Because parents/guardians may express concern about the likelihood of transmitting diseases through human milk, this issue is addressed in detail to assure there is a very small risk of such transmission occurring.

If a child has been mistakenly fed another child's bottle of expressed human milk, the possible exposure to infectious diseases should be treated just as if an unintentional exposure to other body fluids had occurred.

The early care and education program should (1):

a. Inform the mother who expressed the human milk about the mistake and when the bottle switch occurred, and ask:
    1. When the human milk was expressed and how it was handled prior to being delivered to the caregiver/teacher or facility;
    2. Whether the mother has ever had a Human Immunodeficiency Virus (HIV) blood test and, if so, the date of the test and would she be willing to share the results with the parents/guardians of the child who was fed her child's milk;

3. If she does not know whether she has ever been tested for HIV, ask her if would she be willing to contact her primary health care provider and find out if she has been tested; and

4. If she has never been tested for HIV, would she be willing to be tested and share the results with the parents/guardians of the other child.

b. Discuss the mistake with the parents/guardians of the child who was fed the wrong bottle:

1. Inform them that their child was given another child's bottle of expressed human milk and the date it was given;

2. Inform them that the risk of transmission of HIV is low;

3. Encourage the parents/guardians to notify the child's primary health care provider of the potential exposure; and

4. Provide the family with information including the time at which the milk was expressed and how the milk was handled prior to its being delivered to the caregiver/teacher so that the parents/guardians may inform the child's primary health care provider.

c. Assess why the wrong milk was given and develop a prevention plan to be shared with the parents/guardians as well as the staff in the facility.

RATIONALE
Hepatitis B and C are not spread through breastfeeding (2,3).

The risk of HIV transmission from expressed human milk consumed by another child is believed to be low because:

a. Transmission of HIV from a single human milk exposure has never been documented (1);

b. Chemicals present in human milk stored in cold temperatures, act to destroy the HIV present in expressed human milk; and

c. In the United States, women who know they are HIV-positive are advised NOT to breastfeed their infants and to refrain from breastfeeding if they are hepatitis C-positive or have cracked or bleeding nipples. [However, the transmission of hepatitis C by breastfeeding has not been documented (4).]

RELATED STANDARD
Preparing, Feeding, and Storing Human Milk

REFERENCES
1. U.S. Centers for Disease Control and Prevention. 2016. What to do if an infant or child is mistakenly fed another woman's expressed breast milk. http://www.cdc.gov/breastfeeding/recommendations/other_mothers_milk.htm.
2. U.S. Centers for Disease Control and Prevention. 2016. Hepatitis B FAQs for the public. https://www.cdc.gov/hepatitis/hbv/bfaq.htm#bFAQ13.
3. U.S. Centers for Disease Control and Prevention. 2016. Hepatitis C FAQs for the public. https://www.cdc.gov/hepatitis/hcv/cfaq.htm#cFAQ37.
4. Kimberlin, D.W., Brady, M.T., Jackson, M.A., Long, S.S., eds. 2015. *Red Book: 2015 Report of the Committee on Infectious Diseases.* 30th Ed. Elk Grove Village, IL: American Academy of Pediatrics.

NOTES
Content in the STANDARD was modified on 8/24/2017.

Preparing, Feeding, and Storing Infant Formula

Formula provided by parents/guardians or by the facility should come in a factory-sealed container. The formula should be of the same brand that is served at home and should be of ready-to-feed strength or liquid concentrate to be diluted using cold water from a source approved by the health department. Powdered infant formula, though it is the least expensive formula, requires special handling in mixing because it cannot be sterilized. The primary source for proper and safe handling and mixing is the manufacturer's instructions that appear on the can of powdered formula. Before opening the can, hands should be washed. The can and plastic lid should be thoroughly rinsed and dried. Caregivers/teachers should read and follow the manufacturer's directions. Caregivers/teachers should only use the scoop that comes with the can and not interchange the scoop from one product to another, since the volume of the scoop may vary from manufacturer to manufacturer and product to product. Also, a scoop can be contaminated with a potential allergen from another type of formula. If instructions are not readily available, caregivers/teachers should obtain information from their local WIC program or the World Health Organization's Safe Preparation, Storage and Handling of Powdered Infant Formula Guidelines at: http://www.who.int/foodsafety/publications/micro/pif_guidelines.pdf (1).

Formula mixed with cereal, fruit juice, or any other foods should not be served unless the child's primary care provider provides written documentation that the child has a medical reason for this type of feeding.

Iron-fortified formula should be refrigerated until immediately before feeding. For bottles containing formula, any contents remaining after a feeding should be discarded.

Bottles of formula prepared from powder or concentrate or ready-to-feed formula should be labeled with the child's full name and time and date of preparation. Any prepared formula must be discarded within one hour after serving to an infant. Prepared powdered formula that has not been given to an infant should be covered, labeled with date and time of preparation and child's full name, and may be stored in the refrigerator for up to twenty-four hours. An open container of ready-to-feed, concentrated formula, or formula prepared from concentrated formula, should be covered, refrigerated, labeled with date of opening and child's full name, and discarded at forty-eight hours if not used (2). The caregiver/teacher should always follow manufacturer's instructions for mixing and storing of any formula preparation. Some infants will require specialized formula because of allergy, inability to digest certain formulas, or need for extra calories. The appropriate formula should always be available and should be fed as directed. For those infants getting supplemental calories, the formula may be prepared in a different way from the directions on the container. In those circumstances, either the family should provide the prepared formula or the caregiver/teacher should receive special training, as noted in the infant's care plan, on how to prepare the formula. Formula should not be used beyond the stated shelf life period (3).

Parents/guardians should supply enough clean and sterilized bottles to be used throughout the day. The bottles must be sanitary, properly prepared and stored, and must be the same brand in the early care and education program and at home. Avoid bottles made of plastics containing bisphenol A (BPA) or phthalates (sometimes labeled with #3, #6, or #7). Use glass bottles with a silicone sleeve (a silicone bottle jacket to prevent breakage) or those made with safer plastics such as polypropylene or polyethylene (labeled BPA-free) or plastics with a recycling code of #1, #2, #4, or #5.

RATIONALE
Caregivers/teachers help in promoting the feeding of infant formula that is familiar to the infant and supports family feeding practice. By following this standard, the staff is able, when necessary, to prepare formula and feed an infant safely, thereby reducing the risk of inaccuracy or feeding the infant unsanitary or incorrect formula. Written guidance for both staff and parents/guardians must be available to determine when formula provided by parents/guardians will not be served. Formula cannot be served if it does not meet the requirements for sanitary and safe formula.

Staff preparing formula should thoroughly wash their hands prior to beginning preparation of infant feedings of any type. Water used for mixing infant formula must be from a safe water source as defined by the local or state health department. If the caregiver/teacher is concerned or uncertain about the safety of the tap water, s/he should "flush" the water system by running the tap on cold for 1–2 minutes or use bottled water (4). Warmed water should be tested in advance to make sure it is not too hot for the infant. To test the temperature, the caregiver/teacher should shake a few drops on the inside of her/his wrist. A bottle can be prepared by adding powdered formula and room temperature water from the tap just before feeding. Bottles made in this way from powdered formula can be ready for feeding as no additional refrigeration or warming would be required.

Adding too little water to formula puts a burden on an infant's kidneys and digestive system and may lead to dehydration (5). Adding too much water dilutes the formula.

Diluted formula may interfere with an infant's growth and health because it provides inadequate calories and nutrients and can cause water intoxication. Water intoxication can occur in breastfed or formula-fed infants or children over one year of age who are fed an excessive amount of water. Water intoxication can be life-threatening to an infant or young child (6). If a child has a special health problem, such as reflux, or inability to take in nutrients because of delayed development of feeding skills, the child's primary care provider should provide a written plan for the staff to follow so that the child is fed appropriately. Some infants are allergic to milk and soy and need to be fed an elemental formula which does not contain allergens. Other infants need supplemental calories because of poor weight gain.

Infants should not be fed a formula different from the one the parents/guardians feed at home, as even minor differences in formula can cause gastrointestinal upsets and other problems (7).

Excessive shaking of formula may cause foaming that increases the likelihood of feeding air to the infant.

RELATED STANDARDS
General Plan for Feeding Infants
Techniques for Bottle Feeding
Warming Bottles and Infant Foods

REFERENCES

1. World Health Organization. 2007. Safe preparation, storage and handling of powdered infant formula: Guidelines. http://www.who.int/foodsafety/publications/powdered-infant-formula/en/.

2. U.S. Department of Health & Human Services, U.S. Food & Drug Administration. 2016. Food safety for moms to be: Once baby arrives. College Park, MD. https://www.fda.gov/food/resourcesforyou/healtheducators/ucm089629.htm.

3. Seltzer, H. 2012. U.S Department of Health & Human Services. Keeping infant formula safe. https://www.foodsafety.gov/blog/infant_formula.html.

4. Centers for Disease Control and Prevention. 2016. Water. https://www.cdc. gov/nceh/lead/tips/water.htm.

5. Seattle Children's Hospital. 2014. Topics covered for formula feeding: Is this your child's symptoms? Seattle, WA. http://www.seattlechildrens.org/medical-conditions/symptom-index/bottle-feeding-formula-questions/.

6. Brown, J., Krasowski, M. D., & Hesse, M. 2015. Forced water intoxication: A deadly form of child abuse. *The Journal of Law Enforcement*. 4(4).

7. United States Department of Agriculture, Food and Nutrition Service. 2017. *Feeding infants: A guide for use in the child nutrition programs*. https://www. fns.usda.gov/tn/feeding-infants-guide-use-child-nutrition-programs.

NOTES
Content in the STANDARD was modified on 11/5/2013 and 8/25/2016.

Techniques for Bottle Feeding

Infants should always be held for bottle feeding. Caregivers/teachers should hold infants in the caregiver's/teacher's arms or sitting up on the caregiver's/teacher's lap. Bottles should never be propped. The facility should not permit infants to have bottles in the crib. The facility should not permit an infant to carry a bottle while standing, walking, or running around.

Bottle feeding techniques should mimic approaches to breastfeeding:

a. Initiate feeding when infant provides cues (rooting, sucking, etc.);

b. Hold the infant during feedings and respond to vocalizations with eye contact and vocalizations;

c. Alternate sides of caregiver's/teacher's lap;

d. Allow breaks during the feeding for burping;

e. Allow infant to stop the feeding.

A caregiver/teacher should not bottle feed more than one infant at a time.

Bottles should be checked to ensure they are given to the appropriate child, have human milk, infant formula, or water in them. When using a bottle for a breastfed infant, a nipple with a cylindrical teat and a wider base is usually preferable. A shorter or softer nipple may be helpful for infants with a hypersensitive gag reflex, or those who cannot get their lips well back on the wide base of the teat (1).

The use of a bottle or cup to modify or pacify a child's behavior should not be allowed (2).

RATIONALE
The manner in which food is given to infants is conducive to the development of sound eating habits for life. Caregivers/teachers and parents/guardians need to understand the relationship between bottle feeding and emotional security. Caregivers/teachers should hold infants who are bottle feeding whenever possible, even if the children are old enough to hold their own bottle. Caregivers/teachers should promote proper feeding practices and oral hygiene including proper use of the bottle for all infants and toddlers. Bottle propping can cause choking and aspiration and may contribute to long-term health issues, including ear infections (otitis media), orthodontic problems, speech disorders, and psychological problems (3). When infants and children are fed on cue, they are in control of frequency and amount of feedings. This has been found to reduce the risk of childhood obesity. Any liquid except plain water can cause early childhood caries (4). Early childhood caries in primary teeth may hold significant short-term and long-term implications for the child's health (5). Frequently sipping any liquid besides plain water between feeds encourages tooth decay.

Children are at an increased risk for injury when they walk around with bottle nipples in their mouths. Bottles should not be allowed in the crib or bed for safety and sanitary reasons and for preventing dental caries. It is difficult for a caregiver/teacher to be aware of and respond to infant feeding cues when the child is in a crib or bed and when feeding more than one infant at a time. Infants should be burped after every feeding and preferably during the feeding as well.

Caregivers/teachers should offer children fluids from a cup as soon as they are developmentally ready. Some children may be able to drink from a cup around six months of age, while for others it is later (6). Weaning a child to drink from a cup is an individual process, which occurs over a wide range of time. The American Academy of Pediatric Dentistry (AAPD) recommends weaning from a bottle by the child's first birthday (7). Instead of sippy cups, caregivers/teachers should use smaller cups and fill halfway or less to prevent spills as children learn to use a cup (8). If sippy cups are used, it should only be for a very short transition period.

Some children around six months to a year of age may be developmentally ready to feed themselves and may want to drink from a cup. The transition from bottle to cup can come at a time when a child's fine motor skills allow use of a cup. The caregiver/teacher should use a clean small cup without cracks or chips and should help the child to lift and tilt the cup to avoid spillage and left-over fluid. The caregiver/teacher and parent/guardian should work together on cup feeding of human milk to ensure the child's receiving adequate nourishment and to avoid having a large amount of human milk remaining at the end of feeding. Two to three ounces of human milk can be placed in a clean cup and additional milk can be offered as needed. Small amounts of human milk (about an ounce) can be discarded.

RELATED STANDARDS
Feeding Infants on Cue by a Consistent Caregiver/Teacher
Warming Bottles and Infant Foods

REFERENCES
1. Ben-Joseph, E. 2015. Formula feeding FAQs: Getting started. Nemours: KidsHealth. http://kidshealth.org/en/parents/formulafeed-starting.html#
2. Lerner, C., & Parlakian, R. 2016. Colic and crying. Zero to three. https://www.zerotothree.org/resources/197-colic-and-crying.
3. American Academy of Pediatrics, Healthy Children. 2015. Practical bottle feeding tips. https://www.healthychildren.org/English/ages-stages/baby/feeding-nutrition/Pages/Practical-Bottle-Feeding-Tips.aspx.
4. American Academy of Pediatrics, Healthy Children. 2015. How to prevent tooth decay in your baby. https://www.healthychildren.org/English/ages-stages/baby/teething-tooth-care/Pages/How-to-Prevent-Tooth-Decay-in-Your-Baby.aspx.
5. Çolak, H., Dülgergil, Ç. T., Dalli, M., & Hamidi, M. M. 2013. Early childhood caries update: A review of causes, diagnoses, and treatments. Journal of natural science, biology, and medicine, 4(1), 29.
6. Hirsch, L. 2017. Feeding your 4- to 7-month old. Nemours, KidsHealth. http://kidshealth.org/en/parents/feed47m.html#
7. Rupal, C. 2016. Stopping the Bottle. Nemours, KidsHealth. http://kidshealth. org/en/parents/no-bottles.html#.
8. Holt, K., N. Wooldridge, M. Story and D. Sofka. 2011. *Bright futures nutrition*. 3rd ed. Chicago: American Academy of Pediatrics. Print.

Warming Bottles and Infant Foods

Bottles and infant foods do not have to be warmed; they can be served cold from the refrigerator. If a caregiver/teacher chooses to warm them, bottles or containers of infant foods should be warmed under running, warm tap water or by placing them in a container of water that is no warmer than 120°F (49°C). Bottles should not be left in a pot of water to warm for more than 5 minutes. Bottles and infant foods should never be warmed in a microwave oven because uneven hot spots in milk and/or food may burn the infant (1,2).

Infant foods should be stirred carefully to distribute the heat evenly. A caregiver/teacher should not hold an infant while removing a bottle or infant food from the container of warm water or while preparing a bottle or stirring infant food that has been warmed in some other way. Bottles used for infant feeding should be made of the following substances (3):

a. Bisphenol A (BPA)-free plastic; plastic labeled #1, #2, #4, or #5, or
b. Glass (a silicone sleeve/jacket covering a glass bottle to prevent breakage is permissible).

When a slow-cooking device, such as a crock-pot, is used for warming human milk, infant formula, or infant food, the device (and cord) should be out of children's reach. The device should contain water at a temperature that does not exceed 120°F (49°C), and be emptied, cleaned, sanitized, and refilled with fresh water daily. When a bottle warmer is used for warming human milk, infant formula, or infant food, it should be out of children's reach and used according to manufacturer's instructions.

RATIONALE
Bottles of human milk or infant formula that are warmed at room temperature or in warm water for an inappropriate period provide an ideal medium for bacteria to grow. Infants have received burns from hot water dripping from an infant bottle that was removed from a crock-pot or by pulling the crock-pot down on themselves by means of a dangling cord. Caution should be exercised to avoid raising the water temperature above a safe level for warming infant formula or infant food.

ADDITIONAL RESOURCE
Feeding Infants: A Guide for Use in the Child Nutrition Programs, US Department of Agriculture Food and Nutrition Service (https://www.fns.usda.gov/tn/feeding-infants-guide-use-child-nutrition-programs)

RELATED STANDARDS
Preparing, Feeding, and Storing Human Milk
Preparing, Feeding, and Storing Infant Formula
Techniques for Bottle Feeding
Feeding Age-Appropriate Solid Foods to Infants

REFERENCES
1. US Department of Health and Human Services, US Food and Drug Administration. Food safety for moms to be: once baby arrives. https://www.fda.gov/food/resourcesforyou/healtheducators/ucm089629.htm. Updated November 8, 2017. Accessed January 11, 2018
2. Cowan D, Ho B, Sykes KJ, Wei JL. Pediatric oral burns: a ten-year review of patient characteristics, etiologies and treatment outcomes. *Int J Pediatr Otorhinolaryngol*. 2013;77(8):1325–1328

3. Environmental Working Group. Guide to baby-safe bottles and formula. https://www.ewg.org/research/ewg%E2%80%99s-guide-baby-safe-bottles-and- formula#.WlfPqWeWzct. Updated October, 2015. Accessed January 11, 2018

NOTES
Content in the STANDARD was modified on 11/5/2013, 8/25/2016 and 05/31/2018.

Cleaning and Sanitizing Equipment Used for Bottle Feeding

Caregivers/teachers should follow proper handwashing procedures prior to handling infant bottles. Bottles, bottle caps, nipples, and other equipment used for bottle-feeding should be thoroughly cleaned after each use by washing in a dishwasher or by washing with a bottlebrush, soap, and water (1).

Nipples that are discolored, thinning, tacky, or ripped should not be used.

RATIONALE
Infant feeding bottles are contaminated by the infant's saliva during feeding. Formula and milk promote growth of bacteria, yeast, and fungi (2). Bottles, bottle caps, and nipples that are reused should be washed and sanitized to avoid contamination from previous feedings. Excessive boiling of latex bottle nipples will damage them.

ADDITIONAL RESOURCE
Feeding Infants: A Guide for Use in the Child Nutrition Programs, US Department of Agriculture Food and Nutrition Service (https://www.fns.usda.gov/tn/feeding-infants-guide-use-child-nutrition-programs)

RELATED STANDARDS
General Plan for Feeding Infants
Preparing, Feeding, and Storing Human Milk
Feeding Human Milk to Another Mother's Child
Preparing, Feeding, and Storing Infant Formula
Techniques for Bottle Feeding

REFERENCES
1. Centers for Disease Control and Prevention. Water, sanitation & environmentally-related hygiene. How to clean, sanitize, and store infant feeding items. https://www.cdc.gov/healthywater/hygiene/healthychildcare/infantfeeding/cleansanitize.html. Updated April 11, 2017. Accessed January 11, 2018
2. Wolfram T. How to safely clean baby bottles. Academy of Nutrition and Dietetics Eat Right Web site. http://www.eatright.org/resource/homefoodsafety/four-steps/wash/how-to-safely-clean-baby-bottles. Published February 16, 2017. Accessed January 11, 2018

NOTES
Content in the STANDARD was modified on 05/31/2018.

Introduction of Age-Appropriate Solid Foods to Infants

A plan to introduce complementary, age-appropriate solid foods to infants should be made in consultation with the child's parent/guardian and primary health care provider. Complementary foods are foods other than human (breast) milk or infant formula (liquids, semisolids, and solids) introduced to an infant to provide nutrients(1). Age-appropriate solid foods may be introduced at 6 months of age with the flexibility to introduce sooner or later based on the child's developmental status (2). However, recommendations on the introduction of complementary foods provided to caregivers of infants should take into account:
*   The infant's developmental stage and nutritional status
*   Coexisting medical conditions
*   Social factors
*   Cultural, ethnic, and religious food preferences of the family
*   Financial considerations
*   Other pertinent factors discovered through the nutrition assessment process (1)

For infants who are exclusively breastfed, the amount of certain nutrients in the body—such as iron and zinc—begins to decrease after 6 months of age. Therefore, pureed meats/meat substitutes and iron-fortified cereals should be gradually introduced first (3). Iron-fortified cereals, pureed meats, and pureed fruits/vegetables are all appropriate foods to introduce. The first food introduced should be a single-ingredient food that is served in a small portion for 2 to 7 days (3). Gradually increase variety and portion of foods, one at a time, as tolerated by the infant (4). There are several signs that caregivers/teachers should use when determining when the infant is ready for solid foods. These include sitting up with minimal support, proper head control, ability to chew well, or grabbing food from the plate. Additionally, infants will lose the tongue-thrusting reflex and begin acting hungry after formula feeding or breastfeeding (3). Caregivers/teachers should use or develop a take-home sheet for parents/guardians in which the caregiver/teacher records the food consumed, how much, and other important notes on the infant, each day. Caregivers/teachers should continue to consult with each infant's parents/guardians concerning which foods they have introduced and are feeding. When appropriate, modification of basic food patterns should be provided in writing by the infant's primary health care provider.

If nutritional supplements are to be given by caregivers/teachers, written orders from the prescribing health care provider should specify medical need, medication, dosage, and length of time to give medication.

RATIONALE

Early introduction of age-appropriate solid food and fruit juice interferes with the intake of human milk or iron-fortified formula that the infant needs for growth. Age-appropriate solid foods given before an infant is developmentally ready may be associated with allergies and digestive problems (5). Age-appropriate solid foods, such as meat and fortified cereals, are needed beginning at 6 months of age to make up for any potential losses in zinc and iron during exclusive breastfeeding (3). Typically, low levels of vitamin D are transferred to infants via breast milk, warranting the recommendation that breastfed or partially breastfed infants receive a minimum daily intake of 400 IU of vitamin D supplementation beginning soon after birth (6). These supplements are given at home by the parents/guardians, unless otherwise specified by the primary health care provider.

Many caregivers/teachers and parents/guardians believe that infants sleep better when they start to eat age-appropriate solid foods; however, research shows that longer sleeping periods are developmentally (not nutritionally) determined in mid-infancy and, therefore, shouldn't be the sole reason for deciding when to introduce solid foods to infants (7,8). Additionally, for infants who are exclusively formula fed or given a combination of formula and human milk, evidence for introducing complementary foods in a specific order has not been established.

Good communication between the caregiver/teacher and the parents/guardians cannot be overemphasized and is essential for successful feeding in general, including when and how to introduce age-appropriate solid foods.

ADDITIONAL RESOURCE

Feeding Infants: A Guide for Use in the Child Nutrition Programs, US Department of Agriculture Food and Nutrition Service (https://www.fns.usda.gov/tn/feeding-infants-guide-use-child-nutrition-programs)

RELATED STANDARDS

100% Fruit Juice
Written Menus and Introduction of New Foods
Care for Children with Food Allergies
Vegetarian/Vegan Diets
Adult Supervision of Children Who Are Learning to Feed Themselves
Experience with Familiar and New Foods

REFERENCES

1. US Department of Agriculture, Food and Nutrition Service. Special Supplemental Nutrition Program for Women, Infants, and Children (WIC). Chapter 5: Complementary foods. In: Infant Nutrition and Feeding. Washington, DC: US Department of Agriculture; 2009: 101–128 https://wicworks.fns.usda.gov/wicworks/Topics/FG/CompleteIFG.pdf. Accessed January 11, 2018
2. US Department of Agriculture, Food and Nutrition Service. Child and Adult Care Food Program: meal pattern revisions related to the Healthy, Hunger-Free Kids Act of 2010. Final rule. *Fed Regist.* 2016;81(79):24347–24383
3. American Academy of Pediatrics. Working together: breastfeeding and solid foods. HealthyChildren.org Web site. https://www.healthychildren.org/English/ages-stages/baby/breastfeeding/Pages/Working-Together-Breastfeeding-and-Solid-Foods.aspx. Updated November 21, 2015. Accessed January 11, 2018
4. World Health Organization. Infant and young child feeding. http://www.who.int/mediacentre/factsheets/fs342/en. Updated July 2017. Accessed January 11, 2018
5. Abrams EM, Becker AB. Introducing solid food: age of introduction and its effect on risk of food allergy and other atopic diseases. *Can Fam Physician.* 2013;59(7):721–722
6. Thiele DK, Ralph J, El-Masri M, Anderson CM. Vitamin D3 supplementation during pregnancy and lactation improves vitamin D status of the mother-infant dyad. *J Obstet Gynecol Neonatal Nurs.* 2017;46(1):135–147
7. Walsh A, Kearney L, Dennis N. Factors influencing first-time mothers' introduction of complementary foods: a qualitative exploration. *BMC Public Health.* 2015;15:939
8. Robert Wood Johnson Foundation Healthy Eating Research. *Feeding Guidelines for Infants and Young Toddlers: A Responsive Parenting Approach.* Guidelines for Health Professionals. http://healthyeatingresearch.org/wp-content/uploads/2017/02/her_feeding_guidelines_brief_021416.pdf. Published February 2017. Accessed January 11, 2018

NOTES

Content in the STANDARD was modified on 05/31/2018.

Feeding Age-Appropriate Solid Foods to Infants

Caregivers/teachers should thoroughly wash hands prior to serving any foods to infants/children. All jars of baby food should be washed with soap and warm water and rinsed with clean, running warm water before opening. All commercially packaged baby food should be served from a dish and spoon, not directly from a factory-sealed container or jar (1). A dish should be cleaned and sanitized before use to reduce the likelihood of surface contamination.

Age-appropriate solid food should not be fed in a bottle or an infant feeder unless doing so is written in the child's care plan by the child's primary health care provider. Caregivers/teachers should ensure that there are no food safety recalls (2), and examine the food carefully when removing it from the jar to make sure there are no glass pieces or foreign objects in the food. Caregivers/teachers should discard uneaten food left in dishes from which they have fed a child because it may contain potentially harmful bacteria from the infant's saliva (3). If left out, all food should be discarded after 2 hours (4). The portion of the food that is touched by a utensil should be consumed or discarded.

Any food brought from home should not be served to other children. This will prevent cross contamination and reinforce the policy that food sent to the facility is for the designated child only.

Food should not be shared among children using the same dish or spoon.

Unused portions in opened factory-sealed baby food containers or food brought in containers prepared at home should be stored in the refrigerator and discarded if not consumed after 24 hours of storage. Prior to refrigeration, the opened container or jar should be labeled with the child's full name and the date and time the food container was opened.

RATIONALE

Feeding of age-appropriate solid foods in a bottle to a child is often associated with premature feeding (ie, when the infant is not developmentally ready for solid foods) (5,6).

The external surface of a commercial container or jar may be contaminated with disease-causing microorganisms during shipment or storage and may contaminate the food product during removal of food for placement in the child's serving dish.

RELATED STANDARD

Introduction of Age-Appropriate Solid Foods to Infants

REFERENCES

1. Lester J. Nutrition 411: introducing solid foods. Promise powered by Nemours Children's Health System Web site. https://blog.nemours. org/2016/02/nutrition-411-introducing-solid-foods. Published February 22, 2016. Accessed January 11, 2018
2. US Department of Agriculture. Food Safety and Inspection Service Web site. https://www.fsis.usda.gov/wps/portal/fsis/home. Accessed January 11, 2018
3. US Department of Health and Human Services. Baby food and infant formula. Foodsafety.gov Web site. https://www.foodsafety.gov/keep/ types/babyfood/index.html. Accessed January 11, 2018
4. US Department of Health and Human Services, US Food and Drug Administration. Food safety for moms to be: once baby arrives. https://www.fda.gov/food/resourcesforyou/healtheducators/ ucm089629.htm>. Updated November 8, 2017. Accessed January 11, 2018
5. Robert Wood Johnson Foundation Healthy Eating Research. *Feeding Guidelines for Infants and Young Toddlers: A Responsive Parenting Approach.* Guidelines for Health Professionals. http:// healthyeatingresearch.org/wp-content/uploads/2017/02/her_ feeding_guidelines_brief_021416.pdf. Published February 2017. Accessed January 11, 2018
6. US Department of Agriculture Food and Nutrition Service. Feeding Infants: A Guide for Use in the Child Nutrition Programs. Publication FNS-258. Alexandria, VA: US Department of Agriculture; 2017. https:// www.fns.usda. gov/tn/feeding-infants-guide-use-child-nutrition-programs. Accessed January 11, 2018

NOTES

Content in the STANDARD was modified on 05/31/2018.

Use of Soy-Based Formula and Soy Milk

Soy-based formula or soy milk should be provided to a child whose parents/guardians present a written request because of family or religious dietary restrictions on foods produced from animals (ie, cow's milk and other dairy products). Both soy-based formula and soy milk should be labeled with the infant's or child's full name and date and stored properly.

Soy milk should be available for the children of parents/guardians participating in the Special Supplemental Nutrition Program for Women, Infants, and Children (WIC); Child and Adult Care Food Program; or Supplemental Nutrition Assistance Program (SNAP). Caregivers/teachers should encourage parents/guardians of children with primary health care provider—documented indications for soy formula, who are participating in WIC and/or SNAP, to learn how they can obtain soy-based infant formula or soy milk products.

RATIONALE

The American Academy of Pediatrics recommends use of hypoallergenic or soy formula for infants who are allergic to cow's milk proteins (1). Soy-based formula and soy milk are plant-based alternatives to cow's milk, often chosen by parents/guardians due to dietary or religious reasons.

Soy-based formulas are appropriate for children with galactosemia or congenital lactose intolerance (2). Soy-based formulas are made from soy protein isolate with added methionine, carbohydrates, and oils (soy or vegetable) and are fortified with vitamins and minerals (3). In the United States, all soy-based formula is fortified with iron. Soy-based formula does not contain lactose, so it is used for feeding infants with documented congenital lactose intolerance. There are known differences between allergies to cow's milk proteins and intolerance to lactose. The child's specific health concerns (allergy versus intolerance) should be documented by the child's primary health care provider and not based on possible parental/guardian misinterpretation of symptoms.

RELATED STANDARDS

Care for Children with Food Allergies

Vegetarian/Vegan Diets

Preparing, Feeding, and Storing Infant Formula

REFERENCES

1. Greer FR, Sicherer SH, Burks AW; American Academy of Pediatrics Committee on Nutrition and Section on Allergy and Immunology. Effects of early nutritional interventions on the development of atopic disease in infants and children: the role of maternal dietary restriction, breastfeeding, timing of introduction of complementary foods, and hydrolyzed formulas. *Pediatrics.* 2008;121(1):183–191

2. American Academy of Pediatrics. Where we stand: soy formulas. HealthyChildren.org Web site. https://www.healthychildren.org/ English/ages-stages/baby/feeding-nutrition/Pages/Where-We-Stand-Soy-Formulas. aspx. Updated November 21, 2015. Accessed November 14, 2017

3. US Department of Agriculture. Infant feeding guide. WIC Works Web site. https://wicworks.fns.usda.gov/infants/infant-feeding-guide. Modified October 31, 2017. Accessed November 14, 2017

NOTES

Content in the STANDARD was modified on 05/30/2018.

Requirements for Toddlers and Preschoolers

Meal and Snack Patterns for Toddlers and Preschoolers

Meals and snacks should contain the minimum amount of foods shown in the meal and snack patterns for toddlers and preschoolers described in the Child and Adult Care Food Program (CACFP).

When incorporating CACFP, caregivers/teachers should (1):

- Provide a variety of fruits and vegetables.
- Serve a fruit and/or vegetable during scheduled snacks.
- Provide one serving each of dark-green vegetables, red and orange vegetables, beans and peas, starchy vegetables, and other vegetables weekly.
- Serve whole grains and whole-grain products.
- Limit yogurt to no more than 23 grams of sugar per 6 ounces.
- Limit processed foods to once per week.

Flavored milks contain higher amounts of added sugars and should not be served. Facilities are encouraged to incorporate seasonal/locally produced foods into meals. Water should not be offered to children during mealtimes; instead, offer water throughout the day.

With limited appetites and selective eating by toddlers and preschoolers, less nutritious foods should not be served because they can displace more nutritious foods from the child's diet. Early care and education settings should check with state regulators about the timing between meals. State agencies may require any institution or facility to allow a specific amount of time to elapse between meal services or require that meal services not exceed a specified duration (2).

RATIONALE

Following CACFP guidelines ensures that all children enrolled receive a greater variety of vegetables and fruits and more whole grains and less added sugar and saturated fat during their meals while in care (3). Even during periods of slower growth, children must continue to eat nutritious foods. Picky or selective eating is common among toddlers. They may decide to eat a meal/snack one day but not the next. Over time, with consistent exposure, toddlers are more likely to accept new foods (4).

ADDITIONAL RESOURCES

US Department of Agriculture Food and Nutrition Service CACFP Nutrition Standards for CACFP Meals and Snacks (www.fns.usda.gov/ cacfp/meals-and- snacks)

US Department of Agriculture Healthy Tips for Picky Eaters (https:// wicworks. fns.usda.gov/wicworks/Topics/TipsPickyEaters.pdf)

RELATED STANDARDS

Use of US Department of Agriculture Child and Adult Care Food Program Guidelines

Categories of Foods

Meal and Snack Patterns

REFERENCES

1. US Department of Agriculture. Child and Adult Care Food Program: best practices. https://www.fns.usda.gov/sites/default/files/cacfp/ CACFP_factBP. pdf. Accessed January 11, 2018

2. US Department of Agriculture Food and Nutrition Service. Child and Adult Care Food Program: meal pattern revisions related to the Healthy, Hunger-Free Kids Act of 2010. Final rule. Fed Regist. 2016;81(79):24347–24383. https://www.gpo.gov/fdsys/pkg/ FR-2016-04-25/pdf/2016-09412.pdf. Accessed January 11, 2018

3. US Department of Agriculture Food and Nutrition Service. Independent Child Care Centers: A Child and Adult Care Food Program Handbook. Washington, DC: US Department of Agriculture; 2014. https://fns-prod. azureedge.net/sites/default/files/cacfp/ Independent%20Child%20Care%20 Centers%20Handbook.pdf. Accessed January 11, 2018

4. US Department of Agriculture. Updated Child and Adult Care Food Program meal patterns: child and adult meals. https://www.fns.usda.gov/sites/default/files/cacfp/CACFP_MealBP.pdf. Accessed January 11, 2018

NOTES
Content in the STANDARD was modified on 05/31/2018.

Serving Size for Toddlers and Preschoolers

The facility should serve toddlers and preschoolers small, age-appropriate portions. The facility should permit children to have one or more additional servings of nutritious foods that are low in fat, sugar, and sodium as required to meet the caloric needs of the individual child. Serving dishes should contain, at minimum, the amount of food based on serving sizes or portions recommended for each child outlined in the Child and Adult Care Food Program (CACFP). Young children should learn what appropriate portion size is by being served plates, bowls, and cups that are developmentally and age appropriate.

Food service staff and/or a caregiver/teacher is responsible for preparing the amount of food based on the recommended age-appropriate amount of food per serving for each child to be fed. Usually a reasonable amount of additional food is prepared to respond to any spills or to children requesting a second serving.

Children should continue to be exposed to new foods, textures, and tastes throughout infancy, toddlerhood, and preschool. Children should not be required or forced to eat any specific food items. Caregivers/teachers should create a supportive environment that promotes positive, sound eating behaviors (1).

RATIONALE
A child will not eat the same amount each day because appetites vary and food jags are common (2). Eating habits established in infancy and early childhood may contribute to optimal eating patterns later in life. These habits include nutritious meals/snacks consumed in a pleasant, clean, supportive mealtime atmosphere with age-appropriate plates/utensils (1). The quality of snacks for young and school-aged children is especially important, and small, frequent feedings are recommended to achieve the total desired daily intake.

Strong evidence supports that larger plates, bowls, and cups, when paired with sustained long-term exposure of oversized portions, promote overeating (3). Allowing children to decide how much to eat, through

family-style dining, may also help promote self-regulation in children (3).

COMMENTS
The CACFP guidelines for meal and snack patterns can be found at www.fns.usda.gov/cacfp/meals-and-snacks.

RELATED STANDARDS
Use of US Department of Agriculture Child and Adult Care Food Program Guidelines
Meal and Snack Patterns for Toddlers and Preschoolers
Encouraging Self-Feeding by Older Infants and Toddlers

REFERENCES
1. Mita SC, Gray SA, Goodell LS. An explanatory framework of teachers' perceptions of a positive mealtime environment in a preschool setting. *Appetite*. 2015;90:37–44
2. Green RJ, Samy G, Miqdady MS, et al. How to improve eating behavior during early childhood. *Pediatric Gastroenterol Hepatol Nutr*. 2015;18(1):1–9
3. McCrickerd K, Leong C, Forde CG. Preschool children's sensitivity to teacher-served portion size is linked to age related differences in leftovers. *Appetite*. 2017;114:320–328

NOTES
Content in the STANDARD was modified on 05/31/2018.

Encouraging Self-Feeding by Older Infants and Toddlers

Caregivers/teachers should encourage older infants and toddlers to:
• hold and drink from an appropriate child-sized cup,
• use a child-sized spoon (short handle with a shallow bowl like a soup spoon), and
• use a child-sized fork (short, blunt tines and broad handle, similar to a salad fork).

All of which are developmentally appropriate for young children to feed themselves. Children can also use their fingers for self-feeding. Children in group care should be provided with opportunities to serve and eat a variety of food for themselves. Foods served should be appropriate to the toddler's developmental ability and cut small enough to avoid choking hazards.

RATIONALE
As children enter the second year after birth, they are interested in doing things for themselves. Self-feeding appropriately separates the responsibilities of adults and children. The caregivers/teachers and parents/guardians are responsible for providing nutritious food, and the child is responsible for deciding how much of it to eat (1,2). To

allow for the proper development of motor skills and eating habits, children need to be allowed to practice feeding themselves as early as 9 months of age (3,4). Children will continue to self-feed using their fingers even after mastering the use of a utensil.

RELATED STANDARDS
Serving Size for Toddlers and Preschoolers
Numbers of Children Fed Simultaneously by One Adult
Adult Supervision of Children Who Are Learning to Feed Themselves

REFERENCES
1. McCrickerd K, Leong C, Forde CG. Preschool children's sensitivity to teacher-served portion size is linked to age related differences in leftovers. *Appetite*. 2017;114:320–328
2. American Academy of Pediatrics Committee on Nutrition. *Pediatric Nutrition*. Kleinman RE, Greer FR, eds. 7th ed. Elk Grove Village, IL: American Academy of Pediatrics; 2014
3. Williamson C, Beatty C. Weaning and childhood nutrition. *InnovAiT*. 2015;8(3):141–145
4. Fewtrell M, Bronsky J, Campoy C, et al. Complementary feeding: a position paper by the European Society for Paediatric Gastroenterology, Hepatology, and Nutrition (ESPGHAN) Committee on Nutrition. *J PediatrGastroenterol Nutr*.2017;64(1):119–132

NOTES
Content in the STANDARD was modified on 05/31/2018.

Feeding Cow's Milk

The facility should not serve cow's milk to infants from birth to 12 months of age, unless provided with a written exception and direction from the infant's primary health care provider and parents/guardians. Children between 12 and 24 months of age can be served whole pasteurized milk (1). Children 2 years and older should be served low-fat (1%) or nonfat (skim, fat-free) pasteurized milk (1). With proper documentation from a child's primary health care provider, reduced fat (2%, 1%, nonfat) pasteurized milk may be served to those children who are at risk for high cholesterol or obesity after 12 months of age (2).

RATIONALE
Milk provides many nutrients that are essential for the growth and development of young children. The fat content in whole milk is critical for brain development as well as satiety in children 12 to 24 months of age (3). For those children whom overweight or obesity is a concern or who have a family history of obesity, dyslipidemia, or early cardiovascular disease, the primary health care provider may request low-fat or nonfat milk (2).

It is not recommended that children consume cow's milk in place of human (breast) milk or infant formula during the first year after birth (1,4). Some early care and education programs have children between the ages of 18 months and 3 years in one classroom. To avoid errors in serving inappropriate milk, programs can use individual milk pitchers clearly labeled for each type of milk being served.

Caregivers/teachers can explain to the children the meaning of the colored labels and identify which milk they are drinking.

RELATED STANDARDS
Categories of Foods
Care for Children with Food Allergies

REFERENCES
1. Holt K, Wooldridge N, Story M, Sofka D. *Bright Futures: Nutrition*. 3rd ed. Elk Grove Village, IL: American Academy of Pediatrics; 2011
2. Oldfield B, Misra S, Kwiterovich P. Prevention of cardiovascular disease in pediatric populations. In: Wong ND, Amsterdam EA, Blumenthal RS, eds. ASPC Manual of Preventive Cardiology. New York, NY: Demos Medical Publishing; 2015:184–194
3. Singhal S, Baker RD, Baker SS. A comparison of the nutritional value of cow's milk and nondairy beverages. *J Pediatr Gastroenterol Nutr*. 2017;64(5):799–805
4. American Academy of Pediatrics. Why formula instead of cow's milk? HealthyChildren.org Web site. https://www.healthychildren.org/English/ages-stages/baby/feeding-nutrition/Pages/Why-Formula-Instead-of-Cows-Milk.aspx. Updated November 21, 2015. Accessed January 11, 2018

NOTES
Content in the STANDARD was modified on 05/30/2018.

Requirements for School-Age Children

Meal and Snack Patterns for School-Age Children

Meals and snacks should contain, at a minimum, the meal and snack patterns shown for school-aged children in the Child and Adult Care Food Program (CACFP). Children attending facilities for 2 or more hours after school need at least 1 snack. Breakfast, or a morning snack, is recommended for all children enrolled in an early care and education facility or in school. Depending on age and length of time in care, snacks should occur 2 hours after a scheduled meal. Early care and education settings should check with state regulators about the timing between meals. State agencies may require any institution or facility to allow a specific amount of time to elapse between meal services or require that meal services not exceed a specified duration (1,2). The quantity and quality of food provided should contribute toward meeting children's nutritional needs for the day and should not lessen their appetites (3).

RATIONALE

Early childhood is a time of rapid growth that increases the need for energy and essential nutrients to support optimal growth (2). Food intake may vary considerably because this is a time when children express strong food likes and dislikes. The CACFP requirements ensure that children in child care centers for longer than 8 hours (common in military child development centers, for example) are given the appropriate number of meals and snacks to meet individual caloric and nutrient needs (1).

COMMENTS

The CACFP meal and snack pattern guidelines can be found at www.fns.usda.gov/cacfp/meals-and-snacks. Programs serving children during the summer months can find the recommendations of the Summer Food Service Program at https://www.fns.usda.gov/sfsp/summer-food-service-program.

REFERENCES

1. US Department of Agriculture Food and Nutrition Service. Child and Adult Care Food Program: meal pattern revisions related to the Healthy, Hunger-Free Kids Act of 2010. Final rule. Fed Regist. 2016;81(79):24347–24383. https://www.gpo.gov/fdsys/pkg/FR-2016-04-25/pdf/2016-09412.pdf. Accessed January 11, 2018
2. US Department of Agriculture Food and Nutrition Service. Independent Child Care Centers: A Child and Adult Care Food Program Handbook. Washington, DC: US Department of Agriculture; 2014. https://fns-prod. azureedge.net/sites/default/files/cacfp/Independent%20Child%20Care%20 Centers%20Handbook.pdf. Accessed January 11, 2018
3. American Academy of Pediatrics Committee on Nutrition. *Pediatric Nutrition*. Kleinman RE, Greer FR, eds. 7th ed. Elk Grove Village, IL: American Academy of Pediatrics; 2014

NOTES

Content in the STANDARD was modified on 05/30/2018.

Meal Service and Supervision

Socialization During Meals

Caregivers/teachers and children should sit at the table and eat the meal or snack together. Family style meal service, with the serving platters, bowls, and pitchers on the table so all present can serve themselves, should be encouraged, except for infants and very young children who require an adult to feed them. A separate utensil should be used for serving. Children should not handle foods that they will not be consuming. The adults should encourage, but not force, the children to help themselves to all food components offered at the meal. When eating meals with children, the adult(s) should eat items that meet nutrition standards. The adult(s) should encourage social interaction and conversation, using vocabulary related to the concepts of color, shape, size, quantity, number, temperature of food, and events of the day. Extra assistance and time should be provided for slow eaters. Eating should be an enjoyable experience at the facility and at home.

Special accommodations should be made for children who cannot have the food that is being served. Children who need limited portion sizes should be taught and monitored.

RATIONALE

"Family style" meal service promotes and supports social, emotional, and gross and fine motor skill development. Caregivers/teachers sitting and eating with children is an opportunity to engage children in social interactions with each other and for positive role-modeling by the adult caregiver/teacher. Conversation at the table adds to the pleasant mealtime environment and provides opportunities for informal modeling of appropriate eating behaviors, communication about eating, and imparting nutrition learning experiences (1–3,5–7). The presence of an adult or adults, who eat with the children, helps prevent behaviors that increase the possibility of fighting, feeding each other, stuffing food into the mouth and potential choking, and other negative behaviors. The future development of children depends, to no small extent, on their command of language. Richness of language increases as adults and peers nurture it (5). Family style meals encourage children to serve themselves which develops their eye-hand coordination (3–5). In addition to being nourished by food, infants and young children are encouraged to establish warm human relationships by their eating experiences. When children lack the developmental skills for self-feeding, they will be unable to serve food to themselves. An adult seated at the table can assist and be supportive with self-feeding so the child can eat an adequate amount of food to promote growth and prevent hunger.

COMMENTS

Compliance is measured by structured observation. Use of small pitchers, a limited number of portions on service plates, and adult assistance to enable children to successfully serve themselves helps to make family style service possible without contamination or waste of food.

RELATED STANDARDS

Serving Size for Toddlers and Preschoolers
Encouraging Self-Feeding by Older Infants and Toddlers
Nutrition Learning Experiences for Children

REFERENCES

1. U.S. Department of Health and Human Services, Administration for Children and Families, Office of Head Start. 2009. *Head Start program performance standards.* Rev. ed. Washington, DC: U.S. Government Printing Office. http://eclkc.ohs.acf.hhs.gov/hslc/HeadStartProgram/ProgramDesignandManagement/Head Start Requirements/Head Start Requirements/45 CFR Chapter XIII/45 CFR Chap XIII_ENG.pdf.

2. Benjamin, S. E., ed. 2007. *Making food healthy and safe for children: How to meet the national health and safety performance standards—Guidelines for out of home child care programs.* 2nd ed. Chapel Hill, NC: National Training Institute for Child Care Health Consultants. http://nti.unc.edu/course_files/curriculum/nutrition/making_food_healthy_and_safe.pdf.

3. Endres, J. B., R. E. Rockwell. 2003. *Food, nutrition, and the young child.* 4th ed. New York: Macmillan.

4. U.S. Department of Agriculture (USDA). 2002. *Making nutrition count for children—Nutrition guidance for child care homes.* Washington, DC: USDA. http://www.gpo.gov/fdsys/pkg/ERIC-ED482991/pdf/ERIC-ED482991.pdf

5. Pipes, P. L., C. M. Trahms, eds. 1997. *Nutrition in infancy and childhood.* 6th ed. New York: McGraw-Hill.

6. Branscomb, K. R., C. B. Goble 2008. Infants and toddlers in group care: Feeding practices that foster emotional health. *Young Children* 63:28–33.

7. Sigman-Grant, M., E. Christiansen, L. Branen, J. Fletcher, S. L. Johnson. 2008. About feeding children: Mealtimes in child-care centers in four western states. *J Am Diet Assoc* 108:340–46.

Numbers of Children Fed Simultaneously by One Adult

One adult should not feed more than one infant or three children who need adult assistance with feeding at the same time.

RATIONALE

Cross-contamination among children whom one adult is feeding simultaneously poses significant risk. In addition, mealtime should be a socializing occasion. Feeding more than three children at the same time necessarily resembles an impersonal production line. It is difficult for the caregiver/teacher to be aware of and respond to infant feeding cues when feeding more than one infant at a time.

A child may need one-on-one feeding based on age or degree of ability. Feeding more than three children also presents a potential risk of injury and/or choking.

RELATED STANDARDS

Feeding Infants on Cue by a Consistent Caregiver/Teacher
Serving Size for Toddlers and Preschoolers
Encouraging Self-Feeding by Older Infants and Toddlers
Socialization During Meals
Adult Supervision of Children Who Are Learning to Feed Themselves

Adult Supervision of Children Who Are Learning to Feed Themselves

Children in mid-infancy who are learning to feed themselves should be supervised by an adult seated within arm's reach of them at all times while they are being fed. Children over twelve months of age who can feed themselves should be supervised by an adult who is seated at the same table or within arm's reach of the child's highchair or feeding table. When eating, children should be within sight of an adult at all times.

RATIONALE

A supervising adult should watch for several common problems that typically occur when children in mid-infancy begin to feed themselves. "Squirreling" of several pieces of food in the mouth increases the likelihood of choking. A choking child may not make any noise, so adults must keep their eyes on children who are eating. Active supervision is imperative. Supervised eating also promotes the child's safety by discouraging activities that can lead to choking (1). For best practice, children of all ages should be supervised when eating. Adults can monitor age-appropriate portion size consumption.

COMMENTS

Adults can help children while they are learning, by modeling active chewing (i.e., eating a small piece of food, showing how to use their teeth to bite it) and making positive comments to encourage children while they are eating. Adults can demonstrate how to eat foods on the menu, how to serve food, and how to ask for more food as a way of helping children learn the names of foods (e.g., "please pass the bowl of noodles").

RELATED STANDARDS

Encouraging Self-Feeding by Older Infants and Toddlers
Socialization During Meals
Numbers of Children Fed Simultaneously by One Adult

REFERENCE

1. American Academy of Pediatrics, Committee on Injury, Violence, and Poison Prevention. 2010. Policy statement: Prevention of choking among children. *Pediatrics* 125:601–7.

Participation of Older Children and Staff in Mealtime Activities

Both older children and staff should be actively involved in serving food and other mealtime activities, such as setting and cleaning the table. Staff should supervise and assist children with appropriate handwashing procedures before and after meals and sanitizing of eating surfaces and utensils to prevent cross contamination.

RATIONALE

Children develop social skills and new motor skills as well as increase their dexterity through this type of involvement. Children require close supervision by staff and other adults when they use knives and have contact with food surfaces and food that other children will use.

COMMENTS

Compliance is measured by structured observation.

RELATED STANDARD
Socialization During Meals

Experience with Familiar and New Foods

In consultation with the family and the nutritionist/ registered dietitian, caregivers/teachers should offer children familiar foods that are typical of the child's culture and religious preferences and should also introduce a variety of healthful foods that may not be familiar, but meet a child's nutritional needs. Experiences with new foods can include tasting and swallowing but also include engagement of all senses (seeing, smelling, speaking, etc.) to facilitate the introduction of these new foods.

RATIONALE

By learning about new food, children increase their knowledge of the world around them, and the likelihood that they will choose a more varied, better balanced diet in later life. Eating habits and attitudes about food formed in the early years often last a lifetime. New food acceptance may take eight to fifteen times of offering a food before it is eaten (1).

RELATED STANDARDS
Written Menus and Introduction of New Foods
Introduction of Age-Appropriate Solid Foods to Infants

REFERENCE

1. Sullivan, S. A., L. L. Birch. 1990. Pass the sugar, pass the salt: Experience dictates preference. *Developmental Psychology* 26:546–51.

Activities that Are Incompatible with Eating

Children should be seated when eating. Caregivers/ teachers should ensure that children do not eat when standing, walking, running, playing, lying down, watching TV, playing on the computer, participating in arts and crafts projects that do not involve food, or riding in vehicles.

Children should not be allowed to continue to feed themselves or continue to be assisted with feeding themselves if they begin to fall asleep while eating. Caregivers/ teachers should check that no food is left in a child's mouth before laying a child down to sleep.

RATIONALE

Seating children, while they are eating, reduces the risk of aspiration (1–5). Eating while doing other activities (including playing, walking around, or sitting at a computer) limits opportunities for socialization during meals and snacks. Eating while watching television is associated with an increased risk of obesity (6–8). Continuing to eat while falling asleep puts the child at great risk for gagging or choking.

COMMENTS

Staff can role model appropriate eating behaviors by sitting down when they are eating and eating "family style" with the children when possible.

For additional information, see Building Mealtime Environments and Relationships: An Inventory for Feeding Young Children in Group Settings (http://www.cals. uidaho. edu/feeding/pdfs/BMER.pdf).

RELATED STANDARDS
Screen Time/Digital Media Use
Socialization During Meals

REFERENCES

1. Benjamin, S. E., ed. 2007. Making food healthy and safe for children: How to meet the national health and safety performance standards—Guidelines for out of home child care programs. 2nd ed. Chapel Hill, NC: National Training Institute for Child Care Health Consultants. http://nti. unc.edu/course_files/curriculum/nutrition/making_food_healthy_and_ safe.pdf.

2. Lally, J. R., A. Griffin, E. Fenichel, M. Segal, E. Szanton, B. Weissbourd. 2003. Caring for infants and toddlers in groups: Developmentally appropriate practice. Arlington, VA: Zero to Three.

3. Endres, J. B., R. E. Rockwell. 2003. Food, nutrition, and the young child. 4th ed. New York: Macmillan.

4. U.S. Department of Agriculture (USDA). 2002. Making nutrition count for children—Nutrition guidance for child care homes. Washington, DC: USDA. http://www.gpo.gov/fdsys/pkg/ERIC-ED482991/pdf/ERIC- ED482991.pdf.

5. AAP Committee on Injury, Violence, and Poison Prevention. 2010. Policy statement—Prevention of choking among children. http://pediatrics. aappublications.org/content/early/2010/02/22/peds.2009-2862.

6. Briley, M., C. Roberts-Gray. 2005. Position of the American Dietetic Association: Benchmarks for nutrition programs in child care settings. J Am Dietetic Association 105:979–86.

7. Dennison, B. A., T. A. Erb, P. L. Jenkins. 2002. Television viewing and television in bedroom associated with overweight risk among low-income preschool children. Pediatrics 109:1028–35.

8. Mendoza, J. A., F. J. Zimmerman, D. A. Christakis. 2007. Television viewing, computer use, obesity, and adiposity in US preschool children. Int J Behav Nutr Physical Activity 4, no. 44 (September 25). http://ijbnpa. org/content/4/1/44/.

9. Art and Creative Materials Institute. 2010. Safety—what you need to know. http://www.acminet.org/Safety.htm.

10. U.S. Consumer Product Safety Commission (CPSC). Art and craft safety guide. Bethesda, MD: CPSC. http://www.cpsc.gov/cpscpub/pubs/5015. pdf.

NOTES
Content in the STANDARD was modified on 8/25/2016.

Prohibited Uses of Food

Caregivers/teachers should not force or bribe children to eat nor use food as a reward or punishment.

RATIONALE
Children who are forced to eat or, for whom adults use food to modify behavior, come to view eating as a tug-of-war and are more likely to develop lasting food dislikes and unhealthy eating behaviors. Offering food as a reward or punishment places undue importance on food and may have negative effects on the child by promoting "clean the plate" responses that may lead to obesity or poor eating behavior (1–5).

COMMENTS
All components of the meal should be offered at the same time, allowing children to select and enjoy all of the foods on the menu.

REFERENCES

1. U.S. Department of Health and Human Services, Administration for Children and Families, Office of Head Start. 2009. Head Start program performance standards. Rev. ed. Washington, DC: U.S. Government Printing Office. http://eclkc.ohs.acf.hhs.gov/hslc/HeadStartProgram/Program Design and Management/Head Start Requirements/HeadStartRequirements/45 CFR Chapter XIII/45 CFR Chap XIII_ENG.pdf.

2. Kleinman, R. E., ed. 2009. Pediatric nutrition handbook. 6th ed. Elk Grove Village, IL: American Academy of Pediatrics.

3. Murph, J. R., S. D. Palmer, D. Glassy, eds. 2005. Health in child care: A manual for health professionals. Elk Grove Village, IL: American Academy of Pediatrics.

4. Benjamin, S. E., ed. 2007. Making food healthy and safe for children: How to meet the national health and safety performance standards – Guidelines for out of home child care programs. 2nd ed. Chapel Hill, NC: National Training Institute for Child Care Health Consultants. http://nti.unc.edu/course_files/curriculum/nutrition/making_food_healthy_and_safe.pdf.

5. Birch, L. L., J. O. Fisher, K. K. Davison. 2003. Learning to overeat: Maternal use of restrictive feeding practices promotes girls' eating in the absence of hunger. Am J Clin Nutr 78:215–20.

Use of Nutritionist/Registered Dietitian

A local nutritionist/registered dietitian, knowledgeable of the specific needs of infants and children, should work with the on-site food service expert and the architect or engineer on the design of the parts of the facility involved in food service. Additionally, the nutritionist/registered dietitian should work with the food service expert and the early care and education staff to develop and to implement the facility's nutrition plan and to prepare the initial food service budget. The nutrition plan encompasses:

a. Kitchen layout;
b. Food budget and service;
c. Food procurement and food storage;
d. Menu and meal planning (including periodic review of menus);
e. Food preparation and service;
f. Child feeding practices and policies;
g. Kitchen and mealtime staffing;
h. Nutrition education for children, staff and parents/guardians (including the prevention of childhood obesity and other chronic diseases, food learning experiences, and knowledge of choking hazards);
i. Dietary modification plans.

RATIONALE

Efficient and cost-effective food service in a facility begins with a plan and evaluation of the physical components of the facility. Planning for the food service unit includes consideration of location and adequacy of space for receiving, storing, preparing, and serving areas; cleaning up; dish washing; dining areas, plus space for desk, telephone, records, and employee facilities (such as handwashing sinks, toilets, and lockers). All facets must be considered for new or existing sites, including remodeling or renovation of the unit (1–5).

COMMENTS

Nutritionists/registered dietitians assist food service staff/caregivers/teachers in planning menus for meals/snacks consisting of healthy foods which meet CACFP guidelines; ensuring use of age-appropriate eating utensils and suitable furniture (tables, chairs) for children to sit comfortably while eating; addressing any dietary modification needed; providing training for staff and nutrition education for children and their parents/guardians; consulting on meeting local health department regulations and meeting local regulations when using an off-site food vendor. This standard is primarily for Centers.

RELATED STANDARDS

Routine Health Supervision and Growth Monitoring
Written Nutrition Plan
Assessment and Planning of Nutrition for Individual Children
Feeding Plans and Dietary Modifications
Food and Nutrition Service Policies and Plans
Appendix: Nutrition Specialist, Registered Dietitian, Licensed Nutritionist, Consultant, and Food Service Staff Qualifications

REFERENCES

1. Endres, J. B., R. E. Rockwell. 2003. *Food, nutrition, and the young child.* 4th ed. New York: Macmillan.
2. U.S. Department of Agriculture (USDA). 2002. *Making nutrition count for children—Nutrition guidance for child care homes.* Washington, DC: USDA. http://www.gpo.gov/fdsys/pkg/ERIC-ED482991/pdf/ERIC-ED482991.pdf
3. Pipes, P. L., C. M. Trahms, eds. 1997. *Nutrition in infancy and childhood.* 6th ed. New York: McGraw-Hill.
4. Benjamin, S. E., K. A. Copeland, A. Cradock, E. Walker, M. M. Slining, Neelon, M. W. Gillman. 2009. Menus in child care: A comparison of state regulations to national standards. *J Am Diet Assoc* 109:109–15.
5. Kaphingst, K. M., M. Story. 2009. Child care as an untapped setting for obesity prevention: State child care licensing regulations related to nutrition, physical activity, and media use for preschool-aged children in the United States. *Prev Chronic Dis* 6(1).

Food Brought From Home

Nutritional Quality of Food Brought From Home

The facility should provide parents/guardians with written guidelines that the facility has established a comprehensive plan to meet the nutritional requirements of the children in the facility's care and suggested ways parents/guardians can assist the facility in meeting these guidelines. The facility should develop policies for foods brought from home, with parent/guardian consultation, so that expectations are the same for all families (1,2). The facility should have food available to supplement a child's food brought from home if the food brought from home is deficient in meeting the child's nutrient requirements. If the food the parent/guardian provides consistently does not meet the nutritional or food safety requirements, the facility should provide the food and refer the parent/guardian for consultation to a nutritionist/registered dietitian, to the child's primary care provider, or to community resources with trained nutritionists/registered dietitians (such as The Women, Infants and Children [WIC] Supplemental Food Program, extension services, and health departments).

RATIONALE

The caregiver/teacher/facility has a responsibility to follow feeding practices that promote optimum nutrition supporting growth and development in infants, toddlers, and children. Caregivers/teachers who fail to follow best feeding practices, even when parents/guardians wish such counter practices to be followed, negate their basic responsibility of protecting a child's health, social, and emotional well-being.

COMMENTS

Some local health and/or licensing jurisdictions prohibit any foods being brought from home.

RELATED STANDARDS

Written Nutrition Plan
Selection and Preparation of Food Brought From Home
Food and Nutrition Service Policies and Plans

REFERENCES

1. Sweitzer, S., M. E. Briley, C. Robert-Gray. 2009. Do sack lunches provided by parents meet the nutritional needs of young children who attend child care? *J Am Diet Assn* 109:141–44.

2. Contra Costa Child Care Council, Child Health and Nutrition Program. 2006. CHOICE: Creating healthy opportunities in child care environments. Concord, CA: Contra Costa Child Care Council, Child Health and Nutrition Program. http://w2.cocokids.org/_cs/downloadables/cc- healthnutrition-choicetoolkit.pdf.

Selection and Preparation of Food Brought From Home

The parent/guardian may provide meals for the child upon written agreement between the parent/guardian and the staff. Food brought into the facility should have a clear label showing the child's full name, the date, and the type of food. Lunches and snacks the parent/guardian provides for one individual child's meals should not be shared with other children. When foods are brought to the facility from home or elsewhere, these foods should be limited to those listed in the facility's written policy on nutritional quality of food brought from home. Potentially hazardous and perishable foods should be refrigerated and all foods should be protected against contamination.

RATIONALE
Food borne illness and poisoning from food is a common occurrence when food has not been properly refrigerated and covered. Although many such illnesses are limited to vomiting and diarrhea, sometimes they are life-threatening. Restricting food sent to the facility to be consumed by the individual child reduces the risk of food poisoning from unknown procedures used in home preparation, storage, and transport. Food brought from home should be nourishing, clean, and safe for an individual child. In this way, other children should not be exposed to unknown risk. Inadvertent sharing of food is a common occurrence in early care and education. The facility has an obligation to ensure that any food offered to children at the facility or shared with other children is wholesome and safe as well as complying with the food and nutrition guidelines for meals and snacks that the early care and education program should observe.

COMMENTS
The facility, in collaboration with parents/guardians and the food service staff/nutritionist/registered dietitian, should establish a policy on foods brought from home for celebrating a child's birthday or any similar festive occasion. Programs should inform parents/guardians about healthy food alternatives like fresh fruit cups or fruit salad for such celebrations. Sweetened treats are highly discouraged, but if provided by the parent/guardian, then the portion size of the treat served should be small.

RELATED STANDARDS
Nutritional Quality of Food Brought From Home
Food and Nutrition Service Policies and Plans

Nutrition Education

Nutrition Learning Experiences for Children

The facility should have a nutrition plan that integrates the introduction of food and feeding experiences with facility activities and home feeding. The plan should include opportunities for children to develop the knowledge and skills necessary to make appropriate food choices.

For centers, this plan should be a written plan and should be the shared responsibility of the entire staff, including directors and food service personnel, together with parents/guardians. The nutrition plan should be developed with guidance from, and should be approved by, the nutritionist/registered dietitian or child care health consultant.

Caregivers/teachers should teach children about the taste, smell, texture of foods, and vocabulary and language skills related to food and eating. The children should have the opportunity to feel the textures and learn the different colors, sizes, and shapes of foods and the nutritional benefits of eating healthy foods. Children should also be taught about appropriate portion sizes. The teaching should be evident at mealtimes and during curricular activities, and emphasize the pleasure of eating. Caregivers/teachers need to be aware that children between the ages of two- and five- years-old are often resistant to trying new foods and that food acceptance may take eight to fifteen times of offering a food before it is eaten (14).

RATIONALE
Nourishing and attractive food is a foundation for developmentally appropriate learning experiences and contributes to health and well-being (1–13,15). Coordinating the learning experiences with the food service staff maximizes effectiveness of the education. In addition to the nutritive value of food, infants and young children are helped, through the act of feeding, to establish warm human relationships. Eating should be an enjoyable experience for children and staff in the facility and for children and parents/guardians at home. Enjoying and learning about food in childhood promotes good nutrition habits for a lifetime (17,18).

COMMENTS

Parents/guardians and caregivers/teachers should always be encouraged to sit at the table and eat the same food offered to young children as a way to strengthen family style eating which supports child's serving and feeding him or herself (19). Family style eating requires special training for the food service and early care and education staff since they need to monitor food served in a group setting. Portions should be age-appropriate as specified in Child and Adult Care Food Program (CACFP) guidelines. The use of serving utensils should be encouraged to minimize food handling by children. Children should not eat directly out of serving dishes or storage containers. The presence of an adult at the table with children while they are eating is a way to encourage social interaction and conversation about the food such as its name, color, texture, taste, and concepts such as number, size, and shape; as well as sharing events of the day. These are some practical examples of age-appropriate information for young children to learn about the food they eat. The parent/guardian or adult can help the slow eater, prevent behaviors that might increase risk of fighting, of eating each other's food, and of stuffing food in the mouth in such a way that it might cause choking.

Several community-based nutrition resources can help caregivers/teachers with the nutrition and food service component of their programs (16–18). The key to identifying a qualified nutrition professional is seeking a record of training in pediatric nutrition (normal nutrition, nutrition for children with special health care needs, dietary modifications) and experience and competency in basic food service systems.

Local resources for nutrition education include:

a. Local and state nutritionists/RDs in health departments, in maternal and child health programs, and divisions of children with special health care needs;
b. Nutritionists/RDs at hospitals;
c. The Women, Infants, and Children (WIC) Supplemental Food Program and cooperative extension nutritionists/RDs;
d. School food service personnel;
e. State administrators of the Child and Adult Care Food Program;
f. National School Food Service Management Institute;
g. Healthy Meals Resource System of the Food and Nutrition Information System (National Agricultural Library, U.S. Department of Agriculture);

h. Nutrition consultants with local affiliates of the following organizations:
 1. American Dietetic Association;
 2. American Public Health Association;
 3. Society for Nutrition Education;
 4. American Association of Family and Consumer Sciences;
 5. Dairy Council;
 6. American Heart Association;
 7. American Cancer Society;
 8. American Diabetes Association;
 9. Professional home economists like teachers and those with consumer organizations;
 10. Nutrition departments of local colleges and universities.

Compliance is measured by structured observation.

Following are select resources for caregivers/teachers in providing ongoing opportunities for children and their families to learn about food and healthy eating:

a. Brieger, K. M. 1993. *Cooking up the Pyramid: An early childhood nutrition curriculum.* Pine Island, NY: Clinical Nutrition Services.
b. Cunningham, M. 1995. *Cooking with children: 15 lessons for children, age 7 and up, who really want to learn to cook.* New York: Alfred A. Knopf.
c. Goodwin, M. T., G. Pollen. 1980. *Creative food experiences for children.* Rev. ed. Washington, DC: Center for Science in the Public Interest.
d. King, M. 1993. Healthy choices for kids: Nutrition and activity education program based on the US Dietary Guidelines. Levels 1–3 and 4–5. Wenatchee, WA: The Growers of Washington State Apples.

RELATED STANDARDS

Health, Nutrition, Physical Activity, and Safety Awareness
Written Nutrition Plan
Socialization During Meals
Participation of Older Children and Staff in Mealtime Activities
Experience with Familiar and New Foods
Nutrition Education for Parents/Guardians
Food and Nutrition Service Policies and Plans
Appendix: Nutrition Specialist, Registered Dietitian, Licensed Nutritionist, Consultant, and Food Service Staff Qualifications

REFERENCES

1. U.S. Department of Health and Human Services, Administration for Children and Families, Office of Head Start. 2009. Head Start program performance standards. Rev. ed. Washington, DC: U.S. Government Printing Office. http://eclkc.ohs.acf.hhs.gov/hslc/HeadStart Program/Program Design and Management/Head Start Requirements/Head Start Requirements/45 CFR Chapter XIII/45 CFR Chap XIII_ENG.pdf.

2. Hagan, Jr., J. F., J. S. Shaw, P. M. Duncan, eds. 2008. *Bright futures: Guidelines for health supervision of infants, children, and adolescents.* 3rd ed. Elk Grove Village, IL: American Academy of Pediatrics.

3. Story, M., K. Holt, D. Sofka, eds. 2002. Bright futures in practice: Nutrition. 2nd ed. Arlington, VA: National Center for Education in Maternal and Child Health. http://www.brightfutures.org/nutrition/pdf/frnt_mttr.pdf.

4. Wardle, F., N. Winegarner. 1992. Nutrition and Head Start. *Child Today* 21:57.

5. Benjamin, S. E., ed. 2007. Making food healthy and safe for children: How to meet the national health and safety performance standards—Guidelines for out of home child care programs. 2nd ed. Chapel Hill, NC: National Training Institute for Child Care Health Consultants. http://nti.unc.edu/course_files/curriculum/nutrition/making_food_healthy_and_ safe.pdf.

6. Dietz, W., L. Birch. 2008. *Eating behaviors of young child: Prenatal and postnatal influences on healthy eating.* Elk Grove Village, IL: American Academy of Pediatrics.

7. Kleinman, R. E., ed. 2009. *Pediatric nutrition handbook.* 6th ed. Elk Grove Village, IL: American Academy of Pediatrics.

8. Lally, J. R., A. Griffin, E. Fenichel, M. Segal, E. Szanton, B. Weissbourd. 2003. Caring for infants and toddlers in groups: Developmentally appropriate practice. Arlington, VA: Zero to Three.

9. Endres, J. B., R. E. Rockwell. 2003. *Food, nutrition, and the young child.* 4th ed. New York: Macmillan.

10. Stang, J., C. T. Bayerl, M. M. Flatt. 2006. Position of the American Dietetic Association: Child and adolescent food and nutrition programs. *J American Dietetic Assoc* 106:1467–75.

11. Pipes, P. L., C. M. Trahms, eds. 1997. *Nutrition in infancy and childhood.* 6th ed. New York: McGraw-Hill.

12. William, C. O., ed. 1998. *Pediatric manual of clinical dietetics.* Chicago: American Dietetic Association.

13. Tamborlane, W. V., J. Warshaw, eds. 1997. The Yale guide to children's nutrition. New Haven, CT: Yale University Press.

14. Sullivan, S. A., L. L. Birch. 1990. Pass the sugar, pass the salt: Experience dictates preference. *Devel Psych* 26:546–51.

15. Murph, J. R., S. D. Palmer, D. Glassy, eds. 2005. *Health in child care: A manual for health professionals.* Elk Grove Village, IL: American Academy of Pediatrics.

16. Benjamin, S. E., D. F. Tate, S. I. Bangdiwala, B. H. Neelon, A. S. Ammerman, J. M. Dodds, D. S. Ward. 2008. Preparing child care health consultants to address childhood overweight: A randomized controlled trial comparing web to in-person training. *Maternal Child Health J* 12:662–69.

17. Ammerman, A. S., D. S. Ward, S. E. Benjamin, et al. 2007. An intervention to promote healthy weight: Nutrition and physical activity self-assessment for child care theory and design. *Public Health Research, Practice, Policy* 4:1–12.

18. Story, M., K. M. Kaphingst, S. French. 2006. The role of child care settings in the prevention of obesity. *The Future of Children* 16:143–68

19. Dietz, W. H., L. Stern, eds. 1998. *American Academy of Pediatrics guide to your child's nutrition.* New York: Villard.

Health, Nutrition, Physical Activity, and Safety Awareness

Early care and education programs should create and implement written program plans addressing the physical, oral, mental, nutritional, and social and emotional health, physical activity, and safety aspects of each formally structured activity documented in the written curriculum. These plans should include daily opportunities to learn health habits that prevent infection and significant injuries and health habits that support healthful eating, nutrition education, physical activity, and sleep. Awareness of healthy and safe behaviors, including good nutrition, physical activity, and sleep habits, should be an integral part of the overall program.

RATIONALE

Young children learn better through experiencing an activity and observing behavior than through didactic methods (1). There may be a reciprocal relationship between learning and play so that play experiences are closely related to learning (2). Children can accept and follow rules, routines, and guidelines about health and safety when their personal experience helps them to understand why these rules were created. National guidelines for children birth to age 5 years encourage their engagement in daily physical activity that promotes movement, motor skills, and the foundations of health-related fitness (3). Physical activity is important to overall health and to overweight and obesity prevention (4). Healthy sleep habits (e.g., a bedtime routine, an adequate amount of sleep) (5,6) helps children get the amount of uninterrupted sleep their brains and bodies need, which is associated with lower rates of overweight and obesity later in life (7–11).

RELATED STANDARDS

Active Opportunities for Physical Activity
Socialization During Meals
Nutrition Learning Experiences for Children
Nutrition Education for Parents/Guardians
Appendix: Physical Activity: How Much Is Needed?

REFERENCES

1. Stirrup J, Evans J, Davies B. Learning one's place and position through play: social class and educational opportunity in early years education. *Int J Early Years Educ.* 2017;1–18

2. Weisberg D, Hirsh-Pasek K, Golinkoff R, Kittredge A, Klahr D. Guided play: principles and practices. *Curr Dir Psychol Sci.* 2016;25(3):177–182

3. Roth K, Kriemler S, Lehmacher W, Ruf KC, Graf C, Hebestreit H. Effects of a physical activity intervention in preschool children. *Med Sci Sports Exerc.* 2015;47(12):2542–2551

4. US Department of Health and Human Services, US Department of Agriculture. 2015–2020 Dietary Guidelines for Americans. 8th ed. Washington, DC: US Government Printing Office; 2015. https://health.gov/dietaryguidelines/2015/resources/2015-2020_Dietary_Guidelines.pdf. Published December 2015. Accessed November 14, 2017

5. Sivertsen B, Harvey AG, Reichborn-Kjennerud T, Torgersen L, Ystrom E, Hysing M. Later emotional and behavioral problems associated with sleep problems in toddlers: a longitudinal study. *JAMA Pediatr.* 2015;169(6):575–582

6. Kelly Y, Kelly J, Sacker A. Time for bed: associations with cognitive performance in 7-year-old children: a longitudinal population-based study. *J Epidemiol Community Health.* 2013;67(11):926–931

7. Institute of Medicine. Early Childhood Obesity Prevention Policies: Goals, Recommendations, and Potential Actions. Washington, DC: Institute of Medicine; 2011. http://www.nationalacademies.org/hmd/~/media/Files/Report%20Files/2011/Early-Childhood-Obesity-Prevention-Policies/Young%20Child%20Obesity%202011%20Recommendations.pdf. Published June 2011. Accessed November 14, 2017

8. Fatima Y, Doi SA, Mamun AA. Longitudinal impact of sleep on over-weight and obesity in children and adolescents: a systematic review and bias-adjusted meta-analysis. *Obes Rev.* 2015;16(2):137–149

9. Li L, Zhang S, Huang Y, Chen K. Sleep duration and obesity in children: a systematic review and meta-analysis of prospective cohort studies. *J Paediatr Child Health.* 2017;53(4):378–385

10. Anderson SE, Andridge R, Whitaker RC. Bedtime in preschool-aged children and risk for adolescent obesity. *J Pediatr.* 2016;176:17–22

11. Lumeng JC, Somashekar D, Appugliese D, Kaciroti N, Corwyn RF, Bradley RH. Shorter sleep duration is associated with increased risk for being overweight at ages 9 to 12 years. *Pediatrics.* 2007; 120(5):1020–1029

NOTES

Content in the STANDARD was modified on 5/30/2018

Nutrition Education for Parents/ Guardians

Parents/guardians should be informed of the range of nutrition learning activities for children in care provided in the facility. Formal nutrition information and education programs for parents/guardians should be conducted at least twice a year under the guidance of the nutritionist/registered dietitian based on a needs assessment for nutrition information and education as perceived by families and staff. The importance of healthy sleep habits should be incorporated into obesity prevention programming. Informal programs should be implemented during teach-able moments throughout the year.

RATIONALE

One goal of a facility is to provide a positive environment for the entire family. Informing parents/guardians about nutrition, food, food preparation, and mealtime enhances nutrition and mealtime interactions in the home, which helps to mold a child's food habits and eating behavior (1–3). Because of the current epidemic of childhood obesity, prevention of childhood obesity through nutrition and physical activity is an appropriate topic for parents/guardians. Periodically providing families records of the food eaten and progress in physical activities by their children will help families coordinate home food preparation, nutrition, and physical activity with what is provided at the early care and education facility. Nutrition education directed at parents/guardians complements and enhances the nutrition learning experiences provided to their children. Similarly, bedtime routines are an important facet of a child's physical, social, and emotional health and development. Interestingly, sleep time has a bigger effect on children's weight than awake time (4).

COMMENTS

One method of nutrition education for parents/guardians is providing healthy recipes that are quick and inexpensive to prepare. Another is sharing information about access to local sources of healthy foods (eg, farmers' markets, grocery stores, healthier prepared foods and restaurant options). Also, caregivers/teachers can provide parents/guardians ideas for healthy and inexpensive snacks, including foods available and served at parents'/guardians' meetings. Education should be helpful and culturally relevant and incorporate the use of locally produced food. Educate parents/guardians that an early bedtime is defined as 8:00 pm or earlier and is associated with fewer parent/guardian- and teacher-reported incidences and attention-deficit issues (4,5). Decreased sleep duration with accompanying sleep- related issues is associated with impaired social-emotional and cognitive function that can increase risk of childhood/adolescent obesity (6). Nutrition education programs may be supplemented by periodic distribution of newsletters and sharing Web sites and/or materials.

REFERENCES

1. US Department of Health and Human Services, Administration for Children and Families, Head Start Early Childhood Learning and Knowledge Center. Head Start policy & regulations. Subchapter B—the administration for children and families, Head Start program. https://eclkc.ohs.acf.hhs.gov/policy/45-cfr-chap-xiii. Accessed November 14, 2017

2. Hagan JF, Shaw JS, Duncan PM, eds. *Bright Futures: Guidelines for Health Supervision of Infants, Children, and Adolescents.* 4th ed. Elk Grove Village, IL: American Academy of Pediatrics; 2017

3. American Academy of Pediatrics Committee on Nutrition. *Pediatric Nutrition.* Kleinman RE, Greer FR, eds. 7th ed. Elk Grove Village, IL: American Academy of Pediatrics; 2014

4. Anderson SE, Andridge R, Whitaker RC. Bedtime in preschool-aged children and risk for adolescent obesity. *J Pediatr.* 2016;176:17–22
5. Kobayashi K, Yorifuji T, Yamakawa M, et al. Poor toddler-age sleep schedules predict school-age behavioral disorders in a longitudinal survey. *Brain Dev.* 2015;37(6):572–578
6. Bonuck KA, Schwartz B, Schechter C. Sleep health literacy in Head Start families and staff: exploratory study of knowledge, motivation, and competencies to promote healthy sleep. *Sleep Health.* 2016;2(1):19–24

NOTES
Content in the STANDARD was modified on 05/30/2018.

Policies

Food and Nutrition Service Policies and Plans

The facility should have food handling, feeding, and nutrition policies and plans under the direction of the administration that address the following items and assigns responsibility for each:

a. Kitchen layout;
b. Food budget;
c. Food procurement and storage;
d. Menu and meal planning;
e. Food preparation and service;
f. Kitchen and meal service staffing;
g. Nutrition education for children, staff, and parents/guardians;
h. Emergency preparedness for nutrition services;
i. Food brought from home including food brought for celebrations;
j. Age-appropriate portion sizes of food to meet nutritional needs;
k. Age-appropriate eating utensils and tableware;
l. Promotion of breastfeeding and provision of community resources to support mothers.

A nutritionist/registered dietitian and a food service expert should provide input for and facilitate the development and implementation of a written nutrition plan for the early care and education facility.

RATIONALE
Having a plan that clearly assigns responsibility and that encompasses the pertinent nutrition elements will promote the optimal health of children and staff in early care and education settings.

For sample policies see the Nemours Health and Prevention Services guide on best practices for healthy eating at http://www.nemours.org/content/dam/nemours/www/filebox/service/preventive/nhps/heguide.pdf.

RELATED STANDARDS
Written Nutrition Plan
Written Menus and Introduction of New Foods
General Plan for Feeding Infants
Feeding Infants on Cue by a Consistent Caregiver/Teacher
Preparing, Feeding, and Storing Human Milk
Serving Size for Toddlers and Preschoolers
Use of Nutritionist/Registered Dietitian
Selection and Preparation of Food Brought From Home
Nutritional Quality of Food Brought From Home
Nutrition Learning Experiences for Children
Nutrition Education for Parents/Guardians
Appendix: Nutrition Specialist, Registered Dietitian, Licensed Nutritionist, Consultant, and Food Service Staff Qualifications
Appendix: Our Child Care Center Supports Breastfeeding

Infant Feeding Policy

A policy about infant feeding should be developed with the input and approval from the nutritionist/registered dietitian and should include the following:

a. Storage and handling of expressed human milk;
b. Determination of the kind and amount of commercially prepared formula to be prepared for infants as appropriate;
c. Preparation, storage, and handling of infant formula;
d. Proper handwashing of the caregiver/teacher and the children;
e. Use and proper sanitizing of feeding chairs and of mechanical food preparation and feeding devices, including blenders, feeding bottles, and food warmers;
f. Whether expressed human milk, formula, or infant food should be provided from home, and if so, how much food preparation and use of feeding devices, including blenders, feeding bottles, and food warmers, should be the responsibility of the caregiver/teacher;
g. Holding infants during bottle-feeding or feeding them sitting up;
h. Prohibiting bottle propping during feeding or prolonging feeding;

i. Responding to infants' need for food in a flexible fashion to allow cue feedings in a manner that is consistent with the developmental abilities of the child (policy acknowledges that feeding infants on cue rather than on a schedule may help prevent obesity) (1,2);

j. Introduction and feeding of age-appropriate solid foods (complementary foods);

k. Specification of the number of children who can be fed by one adult at one time;

l. Handling of food intolerance or allergies (e.g., cow's milk, peanuts, orange juice, eggs, wheat).

Individual written infant feeding plans regarding feeding needs and feeding schedule should be developed for each infant in consultation with the infant's primary care provider and parents/guardians.

RATIONALE

Growth and development during infancy require that nourishing, wholesome, and developmentally appropriate food be provided, using safe approaches to feeding. Because individual needs must be accommodated and improper practices can have dire consequences for the child's health and safety, the policy for infant feeding should be developed with professional nutritionists/ registered dietitians. The infant feeding plans should be developed with each infant's parents/guardians and, when appropriate, in collaboration with the child's primary care provider.

RELATED STANDARDS

General Plan for Feeding Infants
Feeding Infants on Cue by a Consistent Caregiver/Teacher
Preparing, Feeding, and Storing Human Milk
Feeding Human Milk to Another Mother's Child
Preparing, Feeding, and Storing Infant Formula
Techniques for Bottle Feeding
Warming Bottles and Infant Foods
Introduction of Age-Appropriate Solid Foods to Infants
Feeding Age-Appropriate Solid Foods to Infants
Appendix: Our Child Care Center Supports Breastfeeding

REFERENCES

1. Birch, L., W. Dietz. 2008. Eating behaviors of young child: Prenatal and postnatal influences on healthy eating, 59–93. Elk Grove Village, IL: American Academy of Pediatrics.

2. Taveras, E. M., S. L. Rifas-Shiman, K. S. Scanlon, L. M. Grummer-Strawn, B. Sherry, M. W. Gillman. 2006. To what extent is the protective effect of breastfeeding on future overweight explained by decreased maternal feeding restriction? *Pediatrics* 118:2341–48. P

PHYSICAL ACTIVITY/SCREEN TIME STANDARDS

Introduction

Physical activity and movement are an essential part of the development, learning, and growth of young children. During the first 6 years after birth, infants, toddlers, and preschoolers are learning fundamental gross motor skills and need ample opportunities to practice these skills. To best develop their cognitive, language, motor, and social-emotional skills, infants and toddlers need hands-on exploration and social interaction with trusted caregivers.[1] Recent evidence suggests that children may be more attentive and learn better after periods of activity and movement.[2]

The early years are key for instilling healthy physical activity habits, primarily through active play. Physical activity is crucial to maintain a healthy weight and prevent obesity. It is important for early care and education programs to promote a variety of age-appropriate physical activities so children of all ages and abilities can safely enjoy physical activity. Early development of active lifestyle habits may lead to continuing physical activity in adulthood.[3,4]

Although physical activity is essential to young children's growth and learning, there are potential barriers to daily opportunities for active play. These include concerns for children's safety and time and curricular constraints.[5] Caregivers/teachers may have inadequate knowledge or training about how to integrate these opportunities into the daily program.[6,7]

For all young children, opportunities for unrestricted movement foster physical growth and exploration of the environment,[8,9] whereas excessive media use has been associated with lags in achievement of knowledge and skills, as well as negative effects on sleep, weight, and social-emotional health.[4] For example, among 2-year-olds, research has shown that body mass index increases with greater weekly media consumption.[10] Caregivers/teachers must be aware of the cumulative media exposure children experience within and outside of the early care and education setting as they plan their daily activities.[11–13]

The following physical activity standards, along with a related appendix and other resources (eg, *Physical Activity*

Guidelines for Americans), address age-appropriate opportunities, obstacles, policies, and practices for incorporating a variety of physical activities for children in early care and education programs. The screen time/digital media standard supports the development of sound media practices for young children in early care and education.

REFERENCES

1. American Academy of Pediatrics Council on Communications and Media. Media and young minds. *Pediatrics*. 2016;138(5):e20162591. PMID: 27940793 https://doi.org/10.1542/peds.2016-2591

2. US Department of Health and Human Services. *Physical Activity Guidelines for Americans*. 2nd ed. Washington, DC: US Department of Health and Human Services; 2018. https://health.gov/paguidelines/second-edition/pdf/Physical_Activity_Guidelines_2nd_edition.pdf. Accessed April 25, 2019

3. Cooper AR, Goodman A, Page AS, et al. Objectively measured physical activity and sedentary time in youth: the International Children's Accelerometry Database (ICAD). *Int J Behav Nutr Phys Act*. 2015;12:113 PMID: 26377803 https://doi.org/10.1186/s12966-015-0274-5

4. Lindsay AC, Greaney ML, Wallington SF, Mesa T, Salas CF. A review of early influences on physical activity and sedentary behaviors of preschool-age children in high-income countries. *J Spec Pediatr Nurs*. 2017;22(3):e12182 PMID: 28407367 https://doi.org/10.1111/jspn.12182

5. Hesketh KR, Lakshman R, van Sluijs EMF. Barriers and facilitators to young children's physical activity and sedentary behaviour: a systematic review and synthesis of qualitative literature. *Obes Rev*. 2017;18(9):987–1017 PMID: 28589678 https://doi.org/10.1111/obr.12562

6. Ward S, Blanger M, Donovan D, et al. Association between childcare educators' practices and preschoolers' physical activity and dietary intake: a cross-sectional analysis. *BMJ Open*. 2017;7(5):e013657 PMID: 28559455 https://doi.org/10.1136/bmjopen-2016-013657

7. Gunter KB, Rice KR, Ward DS, Trost SG. Factors associated with physical activity in children attending family child care homes. *Prev Med*. 2012;54(2):131–133 PMID: 22178820 https://doi.org/10.1016/j.ypmed.2011.12.002

8. Hewitt L, Stanley RM, Okely AD. Correlates of tummy time in infants aged 0-12 months old: a systematic review. *Infant Behav Dev*. 2017;49:310–321 PMID: 29096238 https://doi.org/10.1016/j.infbeh.2017.10.001

9. Koren A, Kahn-D'angelo L, Reece SM, Gore R. Examining childhood obesity from infancy: the relationship between tummy time, infant BMI-z, weight gain, and motor development—an exploratory study. *J Pediatr Health Care*. 2019;33(1):80–91 PMID: 30131199 https://doi.org/10.1016/j.pedhc.2018.06.006

10. Wen LM, Baur LA, Rissel C, Xu H, Simpson JM. Correlates of body mass index and overweight and obesity of children aged 2 years: findings from the healthy beginnings trial. *Obesity (Silver Spring)*. 2014;22(7):1723–1730 PMID: 24415528 https://doi.org/10.1002/oby.20700

11. Tandon PS, Zhou C, Lozano P, Christakis DA. Preschoolers' total daily screen time at home and by type of child care. *J Pediatr*. 2011;158(2):297–300 PMID: 20980020 https://doi.org/10.1016/j.jpeds.2010.08.005

12. Taverno Ross S, Dowda M, Saunders R, Pate R. Double dose: the cumulative effect of TV viewing at home and in preschool on children's activity patterns and weight status. *Pediatr Exerc Sci*. 2013;25(2):262–272 PMID: 23502043

13. Downing KL, Hnatiuk J, Hesketh KD. Prevalence of sedentary behavior in children under 2 years: a systematic review. *Prev Med*. 2015;78:105–114 PMID: 26231111 https://doi.org/10.1016/j.ypmed.2015.07.019

Physical Activity

Active Opportunities for Physical Activity

The facility should promote all children's active play every day. Children should have ample opportunity to do moderate to vigorous activities, such as running, climbing, dancing, skipping, and jumping, to the extent of their abilities.

All children, birth to 6 years of age, should participate daily in:

a. Two to 3 occasions of active play outdoors, weather permitting (see Playing Outdoors for appropriate weather conditions)
b. Two or more structured or caregiver/teacher/adult-led activities or games that promote movement over the course of the day—indoor or outdoor
c. Continuous opportunities to develop and practice age-appropriate gross motor and movement skills

The total time allotted for outdoor play and moderate to vigorous indoor or outdoor physical activity can be adjusted for the age group and weather conditions.

Outdoor play

a. Infants (birth–12 months of age) should be taken outside 2 to 3 times per day, as tolerated. There is no recommended duration of infants' outdoor play.
b. Toddlers (12–35 months) and preschoolers (3–6 years) should be allowed 60 to 90 total minutes of outdoor play (1).

These outdoor times can be curtailed somewhat during adverse weather conditions in which children may still play safely outdoors for shorter periods, but the time of indoor activity should increase so the total amount of exercise remains the same.

Total time allotted for moderate to vigorous activities:

a. Toddlers should be allowed 60 to 90 minutes per 8-hour day for moderate to vigorous physical activity, including running.
b. Preschoolers should be allowed 90 to 120 minutes per 8-hour day for moderate to vigorous physical activity, including running (1,2).

Infants should have supervised tummy time every day when they are awake. Beginning on the first day at the early care and education program, caregivers/teachers should interact with an awake infant on his/her tummy for short periods (3–5 minutes), increasing the amount of time as the infant shows he/she enjoys the activity (3).

There are many ways to promote tummy time with infants:

a. Place yourself or a toy just out of the infant's reach during playtime to get him/her to reach for you or the toy.
b. Place toys in a circle around the infant. Reaching to different points in the circle will allow him/her to develop the appropriate muscles to roll over, scoot on his/her belly, and crawl.
c. Lie on your back and place the infant on your chest. The infant will lift his/her head and use his/her arms to try to see your face (3,4).

Structured activities have been shown to produce higher levels of physical activity in young children, therefore it is recommended that caregivers/teachers incorporate 2 or more short, structured activities or games daily that promote physical activity (5).

Opportunities to actively enjoy physical activity should be incorporated into part-time programs by prorating these recommendations accordingly (eg, 20 minutes of outdoor play for every 3 hours in the facility).

Active play should never be withheld from children who misbehave (eg, child is kept indoors to help another caregiver/teacher while the rest of the children go outside) (6). However, children with out-of-control behavior may need 5 minutes or fewer to calm themselves or settle down before resuming cooperative play or activities.

Infants should not be seated for more than 15 minutes at a time, except during meals or naps (5). Infant equipment, such as swings, stationary activity centers, infant seats (eg, bouncers), and molded seats, should only be used for short periods, if used at all. A least-restrictive environment should be encouraged at all times (7).

Children should have adequate space for indoor and outdoor play.

RATIONALE

Time spent outdoors has been found to be a strong, consistent predictor of children's physical activity (8). Children can accumulate opportunities for activity over the course of several shorter segments of at least 10 minutes each (9). Free play, active play, and outdoor play are essential components of young children's development (10). Children learn through play, developing gross motor, socioemotional, and cognitive skills. During outdoor play, children learn about their environment, science, and nature (10).

Infants' and young children's participation in physical activity is critical to their overall health, development of motor skills, social skills, and maintenance of healthy weight (11). Daily physical activity promotes young children's gross motor development and provides numerous health benefits, including improved fitness and cardiovascular health, healthy bone development, improved sleep, and improved mood and sense of well-being (12).

Toddlers and preschoolers generally accumulate moderate to vigorous physical activity over the course of the day in very short bursts (15–30 seconds) (5). Children may be able to learn better during or immediately after these types of short bursts of physical activity, due to improved attention and focus (13).

Tummy time prepares infants to be able to slide on their bellies and crawl. As infants grow older and stronger they will need more time on their tummies to build their own strength (3).

Childhood obesity prevalence, for children 2 to 5 years old, has steadily decreased from 13.9% in 2004 to 9.4% in 2014 (14). Incorporating government food programs, physical activities, and wellness education into child care centers has been associated with these decreases (15).

Establishing communication between caregivers/teachers and parents/guardians helps facilitate integration of classroom physical activities into the home, making it more likely that children will stay active outside of child care hours (16). Very young children and those not yet able to walk, are entirely dependent on their caregivers/teachers for opportunities to be active (17).

Especially for children in full-time care and for children who don't have access to safe playgrounds, the early care and education facility may provide the child's only daily opportunity for active play. Physical activity habits learned early in life may track into adolescence and adulthood, supporting the importance for children to learn lifelong healthy physical activity habits while in the early care and education program (18).

ADDITIONAL RESOURCES

Choosy Kids (https://choosykids.com)

EatPlayGrow Early Childhood Health Curriculum, Children's Museum of Manhattan (www.eatplaygrow.org)

Head Start Early Childhood Learning & Knowledge Center, US Department of Health and Human Services, Administration for Children & Families (https://eclkc.ohs.acf.hhs.gov/physical-health/article/little-voices-healthy-choices)

Healthy Kids, Healthy Future; The Nemours Foundation (https://healthykidshealthyfuture.org)

Nutrition and Physical Activity Self-Assessment for Child Care, Center for Health Promotion and Disease Prevention, University of North Carolina (http://healthyapple.arewehealthy.com/documents/PhysicalActivityStaffHandouts_NAPSACC.pdf)

Online Physical Education Network (http://openphysed.org) Spark (www.sparkpe.org)

RELATED STANDARDS

Health, Nutrition, Physical Activity, and Safety Awareness
Playing Outdoors
Caregivers'/Teachers' Encouragement of Physical Activity
Policies and Practices that Promote Physical Activity
Appendix: Physical Activity: How Much Is Needed?

REFERENCES

1. Henderson KE, Grode GM, O'Connell ML, Schwartz MB. Environmental factors associated with physical activity in childcare centers. *Int J Behav Nutr Phys Act.* 2015;12:43

2. Vanderloo LM, Martyniuk OJ, Tucker P. Physical and sedentary activity levels among preschoolers in home-based childcare: a systematic review. *J Phys Act Health.* 2015;12(6):879–889

3. American Academy of Pediatrics. Back to sleep, tummy to play. HealthyChildren.org Web site. https://www.healthychildren.org/English/ages-stages/baby/sleep/Pages/Back-to-Sleep-Tummy-to-Play.aspx. Updated January 20, 2017. Accessed January 11, 2018

4. Zachry AH. Tummy time activities. American Academy of Pediatrics HealthyChildren.org Web site. https://www.healthychildren.org/English/ages-stages/baby/sleep/Pages/The-Importance-of-Tummy-Time.aspx. Updated November 21, 2015. Accessed January 11, 2018

5. US Department of Agriculture, US Department of Health and Human Services. Provide opportunities for active play every day. Nutrition and wellness tips for young children: provider handbook for the Child and Adult Care Food Program. https://fns-prod.azureedge.net/sites/default/files/opportunities_play.pdf. Published June 2013. Accessed January 11, 2018

6. Centers for Disease Control and Prevention and SHAPE America-Society of Health and Physical Educators. Physical activity during school: Providing recess to all students. 2017. https://www.cdc.gov/healthyschools/physicalactivity/pdf/Recess_All_Students.pdf. Accessed January 11, 2018

7.   Moir C, Meredith-Jones K, Taylor BJ, et al. Early intervention to encourage physical activity in infants and toddlers: a randomized controlled trial. *Med Sci Sports Exerc.* 2016;48(12):2446–2453

8.   Vanderloo LM, Martyniuk OJ, Tucker P. Physical and sedentary activity levels among preschoolers in home-based childcare: a systematic review. *J Phys Act Health.* 2015;12(6):879–889

9.   Hnatiuk JA, Salmon J, Hinkley T, Okely AD, Trost S. A review of pre-school children's physical activity and sedentary time using objective measures. *Am J Prev Med.* 2014;47(4):487–497

10. Bento G, Dias G. The importance of outdoor play for young children's healthy development. *Porto Biomed J.* 2017;2(5):157–160

11. Jayasuriya A, Williams M, Edwards T, Tandon P. Parents' percep-tions of preschool activities: exploring outdoor play. *Early Educ Dev.* 2016;27(7):1004–1017

12. Timmons BW, Leblanc AG, Carson V, et al. Systematic review of physical activity and health in the early years (aged 0–4 years). *Appl Physiol Nutr Metab.* 2012;37(4):773–792

13. Donnelly JE, Hillman CH, Castelli D, et al. Physical activity, fitness, cognitive function, and academic achievement in children: a system-atic review. *Med Sci Sports Exerc.* 2016;48(6):1197–1222

14. Centers for Disease Control and Prevention. Overweight & obesity. Childhood obesity facts. Prevalence of childhood obesity in the United States, 2011–2014. https://www.cdc.gov/obesity/data/childhood.html. Updated April 10, 2017. Accessed January 11, 2018

15. Ogden CL, Carroll MD, Lawman HG, et al. Trends in obesity prevalence among children and adolescents in the United States, 1988–1994 through 2013–2014. *JAMA.* 2016;315(21):2292–2299

16. Taverno Ross S, Dowda M, Saunders R, Pate R. Double dose: the cumulative effect of TV viewing at home and in preschool on children's activity patterns and weight status. *Pediatr Exerc Sci.* 2013;25(2):262–272

17. Society of Health and Physical Educators. Active Start: A Statement of Physical Activity Guidelines for Children From Birth to Age 5. 2nd ed. Reston, VA: SHAPE America; 2009. https://www.shapeamerica.org/standards/guidelines/activestart.aspx. Accessed January 11, 2018

18. Simmonds M, Llewellyn A, Owen CG, Woolacott N. Predicting adult obesity from childhood obesity: a systematic review and meta–analysis. *Obes Rev.* 2016;17(2)95–107

NOTES

Content in the STANDARD was modified on 05/29/2018.

Playing Outdoors

Children should play outdoors when the conditions do not pose any concerns health and safety such as a signifi-cant risk of frostbite or heat-related illness. Caregivers/teachers must protect children from harm caused by adverse weather, ensuring that children wear appropri-ate clothing and/or appropriate shelter is provided for the weather conditions. Weather that poses a significant health risk includes wind chill factor below −15°F (−26°C) and heat index at or above 90°F (32°C), as identified by the National Weather Service (NWS) (1). Child Care Center Directors as well as caregivers/teachers directors should

monitor weather-related conditions through several media outlets, including local e-mail and text messaging weather alerts.

Caregivers/teachers should also monitor the air quality for safety. Please reference Protection from Air Pollution While Children Are Outside for more information.

Sunny weather

a. Children should be protected from the sun between the hours of 10:00 am and 4:00 pm. Protective mea-sures include using shade; sun-protective clothing such as hats and sunglasses; and sunscreen with UV-B and UV-A ray sun protection factor 15 or higher. Parental/guardian permission is required for the use of sunscreen.

Warm weather

a. Children should have access to clean, sanitary water at all times, including prolonged periods of physical activity, and be encouraged to drink water during periods of prolonged physical activity (2).

b. Caregivers/teachers should encourage parents/guardians to have children dress in clothing that is light-colored, lightweight, and limited to one layer of absorbent material that will maximize the evapo-ration of sweat.

c. On hot days, infants receiving human milk in a bottle can be given additional human milk in a bottle but should not be given water, especially in the first 6 months of life. Infants receiving formula and water can be given additional formula in a bottle.

Cold weather

a. Children should wear layers of loose-fitting, light-weight clothing. Outer garments, such as coats, should be tightly woven and be at least water repellent when rain or snow is present.

b. Children should wear a hat, coat, and gloves/mittens kept snug at the wrist. There should be no hood and neck strings.

c. Caregivers/teachers should check children's extremities for normal color and warmth at least every 15 minutes.

Caregivers/teachers should be aware of environmen-tal hazards such as unsafe drinking water, loud noises, and lead in soil when selecting an area to play outdoors. Children should be observed closely when playing in dirt/soil so that no soil is ingested. Play areas should be fully enclosed and away from heavy traffic areas. In addition, outdoor play for infants may include riding in a carriage or stroller.

Infants should be offered opportunities for gross motor play outdoors.

RATIONALE

Outdoor play is not only an opportunity for learning in a different environment; it also provides many health benefits. Outdoor play allows for physical activity that supports maintenance of a healthy weight (3) and better nighttime sleep (4). Short exposure of the skin to sunlight promotes the production of vitamin D that growing children require.

Open spaces in outdoor areas, even those located on screened rooftops in urban play spaces, encourage children to develop gross motor skills and fine motor play in ways that are difficult to duplicate indoors. Nevertheless, some weather conditions make outdoor play hazardous.

Children need protection from adverse weather and its effects. Heat-induced illness and cold injury are preventable. Weather alert services are beneficial to child care centers because they send out weather warnings, watches, and hurricane information. Alerts are sent to subscribers in the warned areas via text messages and e-mail. It is best practice to use these services but do not rely solely on this system. Weather radio or local news affiliates should also be monitored for weather warnings and advisories. Heat and humidity can pose a significant risk of heat-related illnesses, as defined by the NWS (5). Children have a greater surface area to body mass ratio than adults. Therefore, children do not adapt to extremes of temperature as effectively as adults when exposed to a high climatic heat stress or to cold. Children produce more metabolic heat per mass unit than adults when walking or running. They also have a lower sweating capacity and cannot dissipate body heat by evaporation as effectively (6).

Wind chill conditions can pose a risk of frostbite. Frostbite is an injury to the body caused by freezing body tissue. The most susceptible parts of the body are the extremities such as fingers, toes, earlobes, and the tip of the nose. Symptoms include a loss of feeling in the extremity and a white or pale appearance. Medical attention is needed immediately for frostbite. The affected area should be slowly rewarmed by immersing frozen areas in warm water (around 104°F [40°C]) or applying warm compresses for 30 minutes. If warm water is not available, wrap gently in warm blankets (7). Hypothermia is a medical emergency that occurs when the body loses heat faster than it can produce heat, causing a dangerously low body temperature. An infant with hypothermia may have bright red, cold skin and very low energy. A child's symptoms may include shivering, clumsiness, slurred speech, stumbling, confusion, poor decision-making, drowsiness or low energy, apathy, weak pulse, or shallow breathing (7,8). Call 911 or your local emergency number if a child has these symptoms. Both hypothermia and frostbite can be prevented by properly dressing a child. Dressing in several layers will trap air between layers and provide better insulation than a single thick layer of clothing.

Generally, infectious disease organisms are less concentrated in outdoor air than indoor air. The thought is often expressed that children are more likely to become sick if exposed to cold air; however, upper respiratory infections and flu are caused by viruses, and not exposure to cold air. These viruses spread easily during the winter when children are kept indoors in close proximity. The best protection against the spread of illness is regular and proper hand hygiene for children and caregivers/teachers, as well as proper sanitation procedures during mealtimes and when there is any contact with bodily fluids.

ADDITIONAL RESOURCES

The National Weather Service (NWS) provides up-to-date weather information on all advisories and warnings. It also provides safety tips for caregivers/teachers to use as a tool in determining when weather conditions are comfortable for outdoor play (www.nws.noaa.gov/om/heat/index.shtml).

The National Oceanic and Atmospheric Administration (NOAA) Weather Radio All Hazards (NWR) broadcasts continuous weather information 24 hours a day, 7 days a week, directly from the nearest NWR office. As an all-hazards radio network, it is a single source for comprehensive weather and emergency information. In conjunction with federal, state, and local emergency managers and other public officials, NWR also broadcasts warning and post-event information for all types of hazards, including natural (eg, earthquakes, avalanches), environmental (eg, chemical releases, oil spills), and public safety (eg, AMBER alerts, 911 telephone outages). A special radio receiver or scanner capable of picking up the signal is required to receive NWR. Such radios/receivers can usually be found in most electronic store chains across the country; you can also purchase NOAA weather radios online at www.noaaweatherradios.com.

To access the latest local weather information and warnings, visit the NWS at www.weather.gov; for local air quality conditions, visit https://www.airnow.gov.

RELATED STANDARDS

Active Opportunities for Physical Activity
Protection from Air Pollution While Children Are Outside
Caregivers'/Teachers' Encouragement of Physical Activity
Appendix: Physical Activity: How Much Is Needed?

REFERENCES

1. National Weather Service, National Oceanic and Atmospheric Administration. Wind chill safety. https://www.weather.gov/bou/windchill. Accessed January 11, 2018

2. Centers for Disease Control and Prevention. Increasing Access to Drinking Water and Other Healthier Beverages in Early Care and Education Settings. Atlanta, GA: US Department of Health and Human Services; 2014. https://www.cdc.gov/obesity/downloads/early-childhood-drinking-water-toolkit- final-508reduced.pdf. Accessed January 11, 2018

3. Cleland V, Crawford D, Baur LA, Hume C, Timperio A, Salmon J. A prospective examination of children's time spent outdoors, objectively measured physical activity and overweight. *Int J Obes* (Lond). 2008;32(11):1685–1693

4. Söderström M, Boldemann C, Sahlin U, Mårtensson F, Raustorp A, Blennow M. The quality of the outdoor environment influences children's health—a cross-sectional study of preschoolers. *Acta Paediatr.* 2013;102(1):83–91

5. KidsHealth from Nemours. Heat illness. http://kidshealth.org/en/parents/heat.html. Reviewed February 2014. Accessed January 11, 2018

6. American Academy of Pediatrics. Children & disasters. Extreme temperatures: heat and cold. https://www.aap.org/en-us/advocacy-and- policy/aap-health-initiatives/Children-and-Disasters/Pages/Extreme-Temperatures-Heat-and-Cold.aspx. Accessed January 11, 2018

7. American Academy of Pediatrics. Winter safety tips from the American Academy of Pediatrics. https://www.aap.org/en-us/about-the-aap/aap-press-room/news-features-and-safety-tips/Pages/AAP-Winter-Safety-Tips.aspx. Published January 2018. Accessed January 11, 2018

8. American Academy of Pediatrics. Extreme temperature exposure. HealthyChildren.org Web site. https://www.healthychildren.org/English/health-issues/injuries-emergencies/Pages/Extreme-Temperature-Exposure.aspx. Updated November 21, 2015. Accessed January 11, 2018

NOTES

Content in the STANDARD was modified on 8/8/2013 and 05/29/2018.

Protection from Air Pollution While Children Are Outside

Supervising adults should check the air quality index (AQI) each day and use the information to determine whether it is safe for children to play outdoors.

RATIONALE

Children need protection from air pollution. Air pollution can contribute to acute asthma attacks in sensitive children and, over multiple years of exposure, can contribute to permanent decreased lung size and function (1,2).

COMMENTS

The federal Clean Air Act requires that the Environmental Protection Agency (EPA) establish ambient air quality health standards. Most local health departments monitor weather and air quality in their jurisdiction and make appropriate announcements. AQI is usually reported with local weather reports on media outlets or individuals can sign up for email or text message alerts at http://www. enviroflash.info.

The AQI (available at http://www.airnow.gov) is a cumulative indicator of potential health hazards associated with local or regional air pollution. The AQI is divided into six categories; each category corresponds to a different level of health concern. The six levels of health concern and what they mean are:

a. "Good" AQI is 0–50. Air quality is considered satisfactory, and air pollution poses little or no risk.

b. "Moderate" AQI is 51–100. Air quality is acceptable, however, for some pollutants there may be a moderate health concern for a very small number of people. For example, people who are unusually sensitive to ozone may experience respiratory symptoms.

c. "Unhealthy for Sensitive Groups" AQI is 101–150. Although general public is not likely to be affected at this AQI range, people with heart and lung disease, older adults, and children are at a greater risk from exposure to ozone and the presence of particles in the air.

d. "Unhealthy" AQI is 151–200. Everyone may begin to experience some adverse health effects, and members of the sensitive groups may experience more serious effects.

e. "Very Unhealthy" AQI is 201–300. This would trigger a health alert signifying that everyone may experience more serious health effects.

f. "Hazardous" AQI greater than 300. This would trigger a health warning of emergency conditions. The entire population is more likely to be affected.

RELATED STANDARD

Playing Outdoors

REFERENCES

1. Gehring, U., Gruzieva, O., Agius, R., Beelen, R., Custovic, A., Cyrys, J.,Von Berg. (2013). Air pollution exposure and lung function in children: The ESCAPE project. *Environmental Health Perspectives: EHP.* 121(11–12), 1357–1364.

2. Lerodiakonou, D. (2016). Ambient air pollution, lung function, and airway responsiveness in asthmatic children. *The Journal of Allergy and Clinical Immunology.* 137(2), 390.

NOTES

Content in the STANDARD was modified on 8/25/2016.

Caregivers'/Teachers' Encouragement of Physical Activity

Caregivers/teachers should promote children's active play and participate in children's active games at times when they can safely do so. Caregivers/teachers should

a. Lead structured activities to promote children's activities 2 or more times per day.

b. Wear clothing and footwear that permits easy and safe movement (1).

c. Provide prompts for children to be active (2,3). (eg, "Good throw!").

d. Encourage children's physical activities that are appropriate and safe in the setting (eg, do not prohibit running on the playground when it is safe to run).

e. Have orientation and annual training opportunities to learn about age-appropriate gross motor activities and games that promote children's physical activity (2,4).

f. Not sit during active play.

g. Limit screen time and other digital media as outlined in Screen Time/Digital Media Use.

Caregivers/teachers should consider incorporating structured activities into the curriculum indoors or after children have been on the playground for 10 to 15 minutes. Caregivers/teachers should communicate with parents/guards about their use of screen time/digital media in the home.

RATIONALE

Children learn from the adult modeling of healthy and safe behavior. Caregivers/teachers may not be comfortable promoting active play, perhaps due to inhibitions about their own physical activity skills or lack of training. Caregivers/teachers may also assume their sole role on the playground is to supervise and keep children safe, rather than to promote physical activity. Continuing education activities are useful in disseminating knowledge about effective games to promote physical activity in early care and education while keeping children safe (4).

Children exposed to less screen time/digital media in early care and education settings engage in more moderate-to-vigorous physical activity compared with children who are exposed to more screen time (5). This gives caregivers/teachers the opportunity to model the limitation of screen time/digital media use and to educate parents/guardians about alternative activities that families can do with their children (2).

ADDITIONAL RESOURCE

American Academy of Pediatrics Council on Communications and Media. Media and young minds. *Pediatrics*. 2016;138(5):e20162591

RELATED STANDARDS

Screen Time/Digital Media Use
Active Opportunities for Physical Activity
Playing Outdoors
Policies and Practices that Promote Physical Activity
Appendix: Physical Activity: How Much Is Needed?

REFERENCES

1. Henderson KE, Grode GM, O'Connell ML, Schwartz MB. Environmental factors associated with physical activity in childcare centers. *Int J Behav Nutr Phys Act*. 2015;12:43

2. Tandon PS, Saelens BE, Copeland KA. A comparison of parent and childcare provider's attitudes and perceptions about preschoolers' physical activity and outdoor time. *Child Care Health Dev*. 2017; 43(5):679–686

3. Tandon PS, Walters KM, Igoe BM, Payne EC, Johnson DB. Physical activity practices, policies and environments in Washington state child care settings: results of a statewide survey. *Matern Child Health J*. 2017;21(3):571–582

4. Copeland KA, Khoury JC, Kalkwarf HJ. Child care center characteristics associated with preschoolers' physical activity. *Am J Prev Med*. 2016;50(4):470–479

5. Taverno Ross S, Dowda M, Saunders R, Pate R. Double dose: the cumulative effect of TV viewing at home and in preschool on children's activity patterns and weight status. *Pediatr Exerc Sci*. 2013;25(2):262–272

NOTES

Content in the STANDARD was modified on 05/29/2018.

Policies and Practices that Promote Physical Activity

The facility should have written policies for the promotion of indoor and outdoor physical activity and the removal of potential barriers to physical activity participation. Policies should cover the following areas:

a. **Benefits:** benefits of physical activity and outdoor play.

b. **Duration:** Children will spend 60 to 120 minutes each day outdoors depending on their age, weather permitting. Policies will describe what will be done to ensure physical activity and provisions for gross motor activities indoors on days with more extreme conditions (ie, very wet, very hot, or very cold).

c. **Type:** Structured (caregiver/teacher-initiated) versus unstructured activity.

d. **Setting:** provision of covered areas for shade and shelter on playgrounds, if feasible (1).

e. Clothing: Clothing should protect children from sun exposure and permit easy movement (not too loose and not too tight) that enables full participation in active play; footwear should provide support for running and climbing. Hats and sunglasses should be worn to protect children from sun exposure.

Examples of appropriate clothing/footwear include:
a. Gym shoes or sturdy gym shoe equivalent.
b. Clothes for the weather, including heavy coat, hat, and mittens in the winter/snow; raincoat and boots for the rain; and layered clothes for climates in which the temperature can vary dramatically on a daily basis. Lightweight, breathable clothing, without any hood and neck strings, should be worn when temperatures are hot to protect children from sun exposure.

Examples of inappropriate clothing/footwear include:
a. Footwear that can come off while running or that provides insufficient support for climbing (2)
b. Clothing that can catch on playground equipment (eg, those with drawstrings or loops)

If children wear "dress clothes" or special outfits that cannot be easily laundered, caregivers/teachers should talk with the children's parents/guardians about the program's goals in providing physical activity during the program day and encourage them to provide a set of clothes that can be used during physical activities.

Facilities should discuss the importance of this policy with parents/guardians on enrollment and periodically thereafter.

RATIONALE

If appropriately dressed, children can safely play outdoors in most weather conditions. Children can learn math, science, and language concepts through games involving movement (3,4).

Having a policy on outdoor physical activity that will take place on days when there are adverse weather conditions informs all caregivers/teachers and families about the facility's expectations. The policy can make clear that outdoor activity may require special clothing in colder weather or arrangements for cooling off when it is warm. By having such a policy, the facility encourages caregivers/teachers and families to anticipate and prepare for outdoor activity when cold, hot, or wet weather prevails.

The inappropriate dress of a child is often a barrier in reaching recommended amounts of physical activity in child care centers. Sometimes, children cannot participate in physical activity because of their inappropriate clothes. Caregivers/teachers can be helpful by having extra clean clothing on hand (5). Children can play in the rain and snow and in low temperatures when wearing clothing that keeps them dry and warm. When it is very warm, children can play outdoors, if they play in shady areas, and wear sunscreen, sun-protective clothing, and insect repellent, if necessary (6). Caregivers/teachers should have water available for children to mist, sprinkle, and drink while in warmer weather.

COMMENTS

For assistance in creating and writing physical activity policies, Nemours provides several resources and best practice advice on program implementation. Information is available at https://www.nemours.org/service/health/growuphealthy/activity/educators.html.

RELATED STANDARDS
Active Opportunities for Physical Activity
Playing Outdoors
Caregivers'/Teachers' Encouragement of Physical Activity
Appendix: Physical Activity: How Much Is Needed?

REFERENCES
1. Weinberger N, Butler, AG, Schumacher P. Looking inside and out: perceptions of physical activity in childcare spaces. *Early Child Development and Care.* 2014;184(2):194–210
2. Tandon PS, Walters KM, Igoe BM, Payne EC, Johnson DB. Physical activity practices, policies and environments in Washington state child care settings: results of a statewide survey. *Matern Child Health J.* 2017;21(3):571–582
3. Bento G, Dias G. The importance of outdoor play for young children's healthy development. Porto Biomed J. 2017;2(5):157–160. http://dx.doi.org/10.1016/j.pbj.2017.03.003. Accessed January 11, 2018
4. Jayasuriya A, Williams M, Edwards T, Tandon P. Parents' perceptions of preschool activities: exploring outdoor play. *Early Educ Dev.* 2016;27(7):1004–1017
5. Henderson KE, Grode GM, O'Connell ML, Schwartz MB. Environmental factors associated with physical activity in childcare centers. *Int J Behav Nutr Phys Act.* 2015;12:43
6. American Academy of Pediatrics. Choosing an insect repellent for your child. HealthyChildren.org Web site. https://www.healthychildren.org/English/safety-prevention/at-play/Pages/Insect-Repellents.aspx. Updated March 1, 2017. Accessed January 11, 2018

NOTES
Content in the STANDARD was modified on 08/25/2016 and 05/30/2018.

Screen Time

Screen Time/Digital Media Use

Please note: For the purposes of this standard "screen time/digital media" refers to media content viewed on cell/mobile phone, tablet, computer, television (TV), video, film, and DVD. It does not include video-chatting with family.

Screen time/digital media should not be used with children ages 2 and younger in early care and education settings. For children ages 2 to 5 years, total exposure (in early care and education and at home combined) to digital media should be limited to 1 hour per day of high-quality programming,* and viewed with an adult who can help them apply what they are learning to the world around them (1).

Children ages 5 and older may need to use digital media in early care and education to complete homework. However, caregivers/teachers should ensure that entertainment media time does not displace healthy activities such as exercise, refreshing sleep, and family time, including meals.

For children of all ages, digital media and devices should not be used during meal or snack time, or during nap/rest times and in bed. Devices should be turned off at least one hour before bedtime. When offered, digital media should be free of advertising and brand placement, violence, and sounds that tempt children to overuse the product.

Caregivers/teachers should communicate with parents/guardians about their guidelines for home media use. Caregivers/teachers should take this information into consideration when planning the amount of media use at the child care program to help in meeting daily recommendations (1).

Programs should prioritize physical activity and increased personal social interactions and engagement during the program day. It is important for young children to have active social interactions with adults and children. Media use can distract children (and adults), limit conversations and play, and reduce healthy physical activity, increasing the risk for overweight and obesity. Media should be turned off when not in use since background media can be distracting, and reduce social engagement and learning. Overuse of media can also be associated with problems with behavior, limit-setting, and emotional and behavioral self-regulation; therefore,

caregivers/teachers should avoid using media to calm a child down (1).

Note: The guidance above should not limit digital media use for children with special health care needs who require and consistently use assistive and adaptive computer technology (2). However, the same guidelines apply for entertainment media use. Consultation with an expert in assistive communication may be necessary.

RATIONALE

The first two years of life are critical periods of growth and development for children's brains and bodies, and rapid brain development continues through the early childhood years. To best develop their cognitive, language, motor, and social-emotional skills, infants and toddlers need hands-on exploration and social interaction with trusted caregivers (1). Digital media viewing do not promote such skills development as well as "real life".

Excessive media use has been associated with lags in achievement of knowledge and skills, as well as negative impacts on sleep, weight, and social/emotional health. (1). For example, among 2-year-olds, research has shown that body mass index (BMI) increases for every hour per week of media consumed (3).

COMMENTS

Digital media is not without benefits, including learning from high-quality content, creative engagement, and social interactions. However, especially in young children, real-life social interactions promote greater learning and retention of knowledge and skills. When limited digital media are used, co-viewing and co-teaching with an engaged adult promotes more effective learning and development.

Because children may use digital media before and after attending early care and education settings, limiting digital media use in early care and education settings and substituting developmentally appropriate play and other hands-on activities can better promote learning and skills development. Such an activity is reading. Caregivers/teachers should begin reading to children at infancy (4) and facilities should make age-appropriate books available for each cognitive stage of development that can be co-read and discussed with an adult. See the American Academy of Pediatrics'"Books Build Connections Toolkit" at https://littoolkit.aap.org/forprofessionals/Pages/home.aspx for more information. The American Academy of Pediatrics has developed a Family Media Use Plan tool, available at https://www.healthychildren.org/English/media/Pages/default.aspx, which can help

---

* Designed with child psychologists and educators to meet specific educational goals

parents/guardians, caregivers, and families identify healthy activities for each child, and prioritize them ahead of limited digital media use (5).

Caregivers/teachers serve as role models for children in early care and education settings by not using or being distracted by digital media during care hours. In addition, if adults view media such as news in the presence of children, children may be exposed to inappropriate language or violent or frightening images that can cause emotional upset or increase aggressive thoughts and behavior. Caregivers/teachers should be discouraged from using digital media for personal use while actively engaging with and super-vising the children in their care. Instead, opportunities for collaborative activities are preferred.

It is important to safeguard privacy for children on the internet and digital media. Pictures and videos of children should never be posted on social media without parent/guardian consent. Caregivers/teachers should know and follow their program's policy for taking, sharing, or posting pictures and videos.

RELATED STANDARDS
Active Opportunities for Physical Activity
Appendix: Physical Activity: How Much Is Needed?

REFERENCES

1. American Academy of Pediatrics Council on Communications and Media. Media and young minds. *Pediatrics*. 2016;138(5):e20162591. http://pediatrics.aappublications.org/content/pediatrics/138/5/e20162591.full.pdf

2. Reid CY, Radesky J, Christakis D, et al., American Academy of Pediatrics Council on Communications and Media. Children and adolescents and digital media. *Pediatrics*. 2016;138(5):e2016593. http://pediatrics.aappublications.org/content/early/2016/10/19/peds.2016–2593.

3. Wen LM, Baur LA, Rissel C, Xu H, Simpson, JM. Correlates of body mass index and overweight and obesity of children aged 2 years: finding from the healthy beginnings trial. *Obesity*. 2014;22(7):1723–1730.

4. American Academy of Pediatrics. Council on Early Childhood. Literacy promotion: an essential component of primary care pediatric practice. *Pediatrics*. 2014;134(2):1–6. http://pediatrics.aappublications.org/content/early/2014/06/19/peds.2014–1384.

5. American Academy of Pediatrics Council on Communications and Media. Media use in school-aged children and adolescents. *Pediatrics*. 2016;138(5):e20162592. http://pediatrics.aappublications.org/content/138/5/e20162592.

ADDITIONAL RESOURCES

American Academy of Pediatrics Council on Communications and Media. Children and adolescents and digital media. *Pediatrics*. 2016;138(5): e20162593. http://pediatrics.aappublications.org/content/pediatrics/early/2016/10/19/peds.2016–2593.full.pdf.

American Academy of Pediatrics. Media and children communication toolkit. AAP.org Web site. https://www.aap.org/en-us/advocacy-and-policy/aap-health-initiatives/pages/media-and-children.aspx. Accessed October 12, 2017.

Campaign for a Commercial-Free Childhood. Screenfree.org Web site. http://www.screenfree.org/. Accessed October 12, 2017.

Common Sense Education. Commonsense.org Web site. https://www.commonsense.org/education/toolkit/audience/device-free-dinner-educator-resources. Accessed October 12, 2017.

Fred Rogers Center for Early Learning and Children's Media at Saint Vincent College. How am I doing? A checklist for identifying exemplary uses of technology and interactive media for early learning. Fredrogerscenter.org Web site. http://www.fredrogerscenter.org/2014/02/25/how-am-i-doing-checklist-exemplary-uses-of-technology-early-learning/. Updated February 25, 2014. Accessed October 12, 2017.

National Association for the Education of Young Children. Technology and interactive media as tools in early childhood programs serving children from birth through age 8. Position Statement. NAEYC.org Web site. http://www.naeyc.org/files/naeyc/PS_technology_WEB.pdf. January 2012. Accessed October 12, 2017.

NOTES
Content in the STANDARD was modified on 10/12/2017.

United States Department of Agriculture

MyPlate, MyWins: Make it yours

Find your healthy eating style. Everything you eat and drink over time matters and can help you be healthier now and in the future.

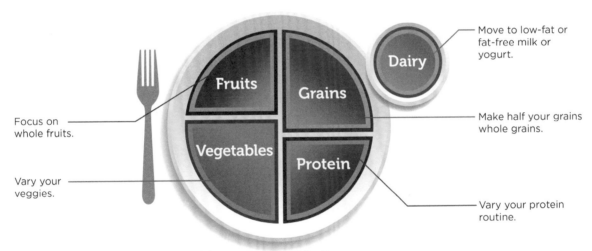

Move to low-fat or fat-free milk or yogurt.

Focus on whole fruits.

Make half your grains whole grains.

Vary your veggies.

Vary your protein routine.

Choose**MyPlate**.gov

Limit the extras.

Drink and eat beverages and food with less sodium, saturated fat, and added sugars.

Create 'MyWins' that fit your healthy eating style.

Start with small changes that you can enjoy, like having an extra piece of fruit today.

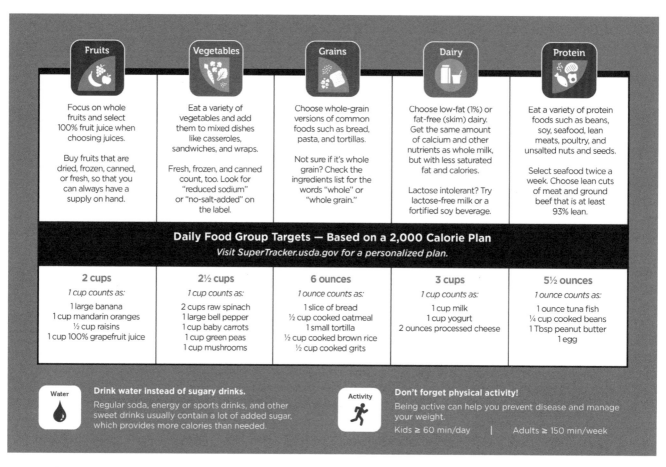

Fruits	Vegetables	Grains	Dairy	Protein
Focus on whole fruits and select 100% fruit juice when choosing juices.

Buy fruits that are dried, frozen, canned, or fresh, so that you can always have a supply on hand. | Eat a variety of vegetables and add them to mixed dishes like casseroles, sandwiches, and wraps.

Fresh, frozen, and canned count, too. Look for "reduced sodium" or "no-salt-added" on the label. | Choose whole-grain versions of common foods such as bread, pasta, and tortillas.

Not sure if it's whole grain? Check the ingredients list for the words "whole" or "whole grain." | Choose low-fat (1%) or fat-free (skim) dairy. Get the same amount of calcium and other nutrients as whole milk, but with less saturated fat and calories.

Lactose intolerant? Try lactose-free milk or a fortified soy beverage. | Eat a variety of protein foods such as beans, soy, seafood, lean meats, poultry, and unsalted nuts and seeds.

Select seafood twice a week. Choose lean cuts of meat and ground beef that is at least 93% lean. |

Daily Food Group Targets — Based on a 2,000 Calorie Plan
Visit SuperTracker.usda.gov for a personalized plan.

2 cups	2½ cups	6 ounces	3 cups	5½ ounces
1 cup counts as:	*1 cup counts as:*	*1 ounce counts as:*	*1 cup counts as:*	*1 ounce counts as:*
1 large banana
1 cup mandarin oranges
½ cup raisins
1 cup 100% grapefruit juice	2 cups raw spinach
1 large bell pepper
1 cup baby carrots
1 cup green peas
1 cup mushrooms	1 slice of bread
½ cup cooked oatmeal
1 small tortilla
½ cup cooked brown rice
½ cup cooked grits	1 cup milk
1 cup yogurt
2 ounces processed cheese	1 ounce tuna fish
¼ cup cooked beans
1 Tbsp peanut butter
1 egg

Water — **Drink water instead of sugary drinks.**
Regular soda, energy or sports drinks, and other sweet drinks usually contain a lot of added sugar, which provides more calories than needed.

Activity — **Don't forget physical activity!**
Being active can help you prevent disease and manage your weight.
Kids ≥ 60 min/day | Adults ≥ 150 min/week

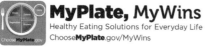

MyPlate, MyWins
Healthy Eating Solutions for Everyday Life
ChooseMyPlate.gov/MyWins

Center for Nutrition Policy and Promotion
May 2016
CNPP-29
USDA is an equal opportunity provider, employer, and lender.

Source
US Department of Agriculture. Choose MyPlate. https://choosemyplate-prod.azureedge.net/sites/default/files/tentips/mini_poster.pdf]. Accessed April 25, 2019

United States Department of Agriculture

10 tips
Nutrition
Education Series

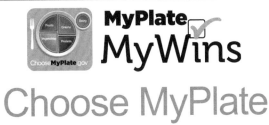

Based on the
**Dietary
Guidelines
for Americans**

Choose MyPlate

Use MyPlate to build your healthy eating style and maintain it for a lifetime. Choose foods and beverages from each MyPlate food group. Make sure your choices are limited in sodium, saturated fat, and added sugars. Start with small changes to make healthier choices you can enjoy.

1 Find your healthy eating style
Creating a healthy style means regularly eating a variety of foods to get the nutrients and calories you need. MyPlate's tips help you create your own healthy eating solutions—"MyWins."

2 Make half your plate fruits and vegetables
Eating colorful fruits and vegetables is important because they provide vitamins and minerals and most are low in calories.

3 Focus on whole fruits
Choose whole fruits—fresh, frozen, dried, or canned in 100% juice. Enjoy fruit with meals, as snacks, or as a dessert.

Fruits

4 Vary your veggies
Try adding fresh, frozen, or canned vegetables to salads, sides, and main dishes. Choose a variety of colorful vegetables prepared in healthful ways: steamed, sauteed, roasted, or raw.

Vegetables

5 Make half your grains whole grains
Look for whole grains listed first or second on the ingredients list—try oatmeal, popcorn, whole-grain bread, and brown rice. Limit grain-based desserts and snacks, such as cakes, cookies, and pastries.

Grains

6 Move to low-fat or fat-free milk or yogurt
Choose low-fat or fat-free milk, yogurt, and soy beverages (soymilk) to cut back on saturated fat. Replace sour cream, cream, and regular cheese with low-fat yogurt, milk, and cheese.

Dairy

7 Vary your protein routine
Mix up your protein foods to include seafood, beans and peas, unsalted nuts and seeds, soy products, eggs, and lean meats and poultry. Try main dishes made with beans or seafood like tuna salad or bean chili.

Protein

8 Drink and eat beverages and food with less sodium, saturated fat, and added sugars
Use the Nutrition Facts label and ingredients list to limit items high in sodium, saturated fat, and added sugars. Choose vegetable oils instead of butter, and oil-based sauces and dips instead of ones with butter, cream, or cheese.

Limit

9 Drink water instead of sugary drinks
Water is calorie-free. Non-diet soda, energy or sports drinks, and other sugar-sweetened drinks contain a lot of calories from added sugars and have few nutrients.

10 Everything you eat and drink matters
The right mix of foods can help you be healthier now and into the future. Turn small changes into your "MyPlate, MyWins."

Center for Nutrition Policy and Promotion
USDA is an equal opportunity provider, employer, and lender.

Go to **ChooseMyPlate**.gov
for more information.

DG TipSheet No. 1
June 2011
Revised October 2016

Source
US Department of Agriculture. Choose MyPlate. https://www.choosemyplate.gov/ten-tips-choose-myplate. Updated July 18, 2017. Accessed April 25, 2019

Physical Activity: How Much Is Needed?

Young Children (2 to 5 years)

Children ages two to five years should play actively, in-short bursts,[1] throughout the day to allow for proper growth and development.[2,3] Caregivers/teachers should encourage free and structured active play that includes a variety of activities (e.g., jumping, tumbling, organized games) that are developmentally appropriate and fun for all children. Total physical activity, light, moderate or vigorous, for this age group may be as much as three hours per day.[3]

Children (6 years and older)

Children should engage in 60 or more minutes of at least moderate physical activity each day.[2] These activities should include a variety of fun, age-appropriate activities that strengthen muscles and bones (e.g., climbing and jumping). Short bursts of activity over the course of a day can accumulate to address the recommended amount of total physical activity.[1,2]

Age-Appropriate Physical Activities

Young children strengthen their muscles by playing outside, climbing on playground structures, or participating in sports such as gymnastics. It is important for early care and education programs to promote a variety of age-appropriate physical activities for children of all ages, beginning with tummy time for infants,[4] and for children of all abilities,[5,6] so they can safely experience daily physical activity. Many physical activities fall into several categories (moderate- and vigorous-intensity and muscle- and bone-strengthening), making it possible for children to gain multiple health-related benefits when early care and education programs incorporate each type of activity. This may increase the chance of children sustaining physical activity into adulthood.[7]

REFERENCES

1. Tucker P. The physical activity levels of preschool-aged children: a systematic review. *Early Child Res Q*. 2008;23:547–58., https://doi.org/10.1016/j.ecresq.2008.08.005. Accessed March 21, 2019.

2. United States Department of Agriculture. *Physical activity: How much is needed?* https://www.choosemyplate.gov/physical-activity-amount. Updated June 21st 2016. Accessed March 8, 2019.

3. U.S. Department of Health and Human Services. *Physical Activity Guidelines for Americans*, 2nd edition. Washington, DC: U.S. Department of Health and Human Services; 2018. https://health.gov/paguidelines /second-edition/pdf/Physical_Activity_Guidelines_2nd_edition.pdf. Accessed March 8, 2019.

4. Hagan JF, Shaw JS, Duncan PM. *Bright Futures: Guidelines for Health Supervision of Infants, Children and Adolescents*. 4th ed. Elk Grove Village, IL: American Academy of Pediatrics; 2017.

5. Shields N, Synnot AJ, Barr M. Perceived barriers andfacilitators to physical activity for children with disability: a systematic review. *Br J Sports Med*. 2012 Nov;46(14):989-97. doi: 10.1136/bjsports-2011-090236.

6. Shields N, Synnot A. Perceived barriers and facilitators to participation in physical activity for children with disability: a qualitative study. *BMC Pediatr*. 2016 Jan 19;16:9. doi: 10.1186/s12887-016-0544-7.

7. Goldfield GS, Harvey A, Grattan K, Adamo KB. Physical activity promotion in the preschool years: a critical period to intervene. *Int J Environ Res Public Health*. 2012;9(4):1326-42. doi: 10.3390/ijerph9041326.

*Because we are committed to
healthy mothers and children,*

Our Child Care Center Supports Breastfeeding

In order to support families who are breastfeeding or who are considering breastfeeding, we strive to do the following:

- Make a commitment to the importance of breastfeeding, especially exclusive breastfeeding, and proudly share this commitment with our staff and clients.

- Train all staff in supporting the best infant and young child feeding.

- Inform families about the importance of breastfeeding.

- Develop a breastfeeding-friendly feeding plan with each family.

- Train all staff to handle, store, and feed mother's milk properly.

- Teach our clients to properly store and label their milk for child care center use.

- Provide a breastfeeding-friendly environment, welcoming mothers to nurse their babies at our center.

- Display posters and brochures that support breastfeeding and show best practices.

- Contact and coordinate with local skilled breastfeeding support and actively refer.

- Continually update our information and learning about breastfeeding support.

Breastfeeding Families Welcome Here!

**Breastfeeding-Friendly
Child Care Initiative**
*A collaboration between
Wake County's Child Care Health
Consultants and the Carolina Global
Breastfeeding Institute*

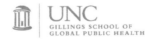

 *Child Care Health
Consultant Program is
funded by Wake County
SmartStart, working to
ensure children, ages 0 to 5,
are prepared for success in
school and in life.*

Nutrition Specialist, Registered Dietitian, Licensed Nutritionist, Consultant, and Food Service Staff Qualifications		
TITLE	**LEVEL OF PROFESSIONAL RESPONSIBILITY**	**EDUCATION AND EXPERIENCE**
Registered Dietitian (State and Local Levels) Licensed Dietitian Nutrition Specialist Nutritionist Child Care Nutrition Consultant	Develops Food/Nutrition policies and procedures and provides consultation to state agency personnel, including staff involved with licensure. Provides expertise to early care and education program directors and provides ongoing guidance, consultation, and staff in-service training.	• Registration with the Commission on Dietetic Registration of the Academy of Nutrition and Dietetics — State licensure required in some states • **OR** A Master's degree from an approved program in public health nutrition may be substituted for registration with the Commission on Dietetic Registration. Current state licensure or certification as a nutritionist or dietitian is acceptable • Two years of related experience as a nutritionist or dietitian in a health program including services in infants and children
Food Service Manager	Oversees the preparation, presentation and delivery of food within an early care and education program.	• High school diploma or GED • Two years of food service experience • Successful completion of a food safety class **OR** experience/coursework in basic menu-planning skills, basic foods, and/or other relevant courses
Food Service Worker (Cook)	Under the supervision of the Food Service Manager, carries out food service operations including menu planning, food preparation and service, and related duties in a designated area.	• High school diploma or GED • One year of food service experience • Successful completion of a food safety class **OR** experience/coursework in basic menu-planning skills, basic foods, and/or other relevant courses
Food Service Aide	Works no more than four hours a day, under the supervision of an employee at a higher level in food service unit.	• High school diploma or GED • Successful completion of a food safety class within one to two months of employment • No prior experience is required

ACRONYMS/ABBREVIATIONS

AAFP — American Academy of Family Physicians

AAP — American Academy of Pediatrics

AAPD — American Academy of Pediatric Dentistry

ABM — Academy of Breastfeeding Medicine

ACS — American Cancer Society

ADA — American Diabetes Association

ADA — American Dietetic Association

AHA — American Heart Association

AIDS — Acquired Immunodeficiency Syndrome

APHA — American Public Health Association

BMI — Body Mass Index

BPA — Bisphenol A

CACFP — Child and Adult Care Food Program

CCHC — Child Care Health Consultant

CDC — Centers for Disease Control and Prevention

CFOC — *Caring for Our Children: National Health and Safety Performance Standards; Guidelines for Early Care and Education Programs*

CFR — Code of Federal Regulations

CSHCN — Children with Special Health Care Needs

EMS — Emergency Medical Services

EPA — U.S. Environmental Protection Agency

FDA — U.S. Food and Drug Administration

HBV — Hepatitis B Virus

HCV — Hepatitis C Virus

HIV — Human Immunodeficiency Virus

HMRS — Healthy Meals Resource System

HRSA — U.S. Health Resources and Services Administration

IU — International units

MCHB — Maternal and Child Health Bureau

NAP–SACC — Nutrition and Physical Activity Self-assessment for Child Care

NASPE — National Association for Sport and Physical Education

NEC — Necrotizing enterocolitis

NFSMI — National Food Service Management Institute

NRC — National Resource Center for Health and Safety in Child Care and Early Education

NWS — National Weather Service

OSHA — Occupational Safety and Health Administration

PBDE — Polybrominated diphenyl ethers

PC — Polycarbonate

PCO3 — *Preventing Childhood Obesity in Early Care and Education Programs,* 3rd ed

SIDS — Sudden infant death syndrome

SNE — Society for Nutrition Education

UNICEF — United Nations Children's Fund

USBC — United States Breastfeeding Committee

USDA — U.S. Department of Agriculture

WHO — World Health Organization

WIC — Women, Infants, and Children

GLOSSARY

See also Acronyms/Abbreviations (page 59).

Note: Some of these definitions were contained in the first edition of *Caring for Our Children* in which they were reprinted with permission from Infectious Diseases in Child Care Settings: Information for Directors, Caregivers, and Parents or Guardians, by the Epidemiology Departments of Hennepin County Community Health, St. Paul Division of Public Health, Minnesota Department of Health, Washington County Public Health, and Bloomington Division of Health. Other definitions are from the resources referenced at the end of the definition. Others were supplied by our Technical Panels.

Aflatoxin — A naturally occurring mycotoxin (fungus) produced by mold. The mold occurs in soil, decaying vegetation, hay, and grains undergoing microbiological deterioration. Favorable conditions include high moisture content and high temperature (USDA).

Age-appropriate solid foods — Also known as complementary foods, foods introduced at age-appropriate levels to infants. Examples are iron-fortified infant cereals and pureed meats for infants.

Allergens — A substance (food, pollen, pets, mold, medication, etc.) that causes an allergic reaction.

Anaphylaxis — A fungus that is most commonly found in corn, cotton, peanuts, and tree nuts. Moisture, insects, and high temperatures can cause aflatoxin crop damage. Growth is most commonly found when a period of drought is followed by a period of high humidity. Aflatoxin can also attack crops during storage or if drying is delayed. Rodents and insects can also cause contamination. Ref: U.S. Department of Agriculture, Risk Management Agency. 2008. A Risk Management Agency fact sheet: Loss adjustment procedures for aflatoxin. Rev. ed. http://www.rma.usda.gov/pubs/rme/aflatoxinfactsheet.pdf

Anemia — Having too little hemoglobin (hemoglobin carries oxygen from the lungs throughout the body). The terms anemia, iron deficiency, and iron deficiency anemia often are used interchangeably. Iron deficiency ranges from depleted iron stores without functional or health impairment to iron deficiency with anemia, which affects the functioning of several organ systems. Ref: Centers for Disease Control and Prevention. 2007. Iron deficiency. http://www.cdc.gov/nutrition/everyone/basics/vitamins/iron.html.

Aspiration — The inhalation of food, liquid, or a foreign body into a person's airway, possibly resulting in choking and respiratory distress.

Assessment — An in-depth appraisal conducted to diagnose a condition or determine the importance or value of a procedure.

Bacteria (Plural of bacterium) — Organisms that may be responsible for localized or generalized diseases and can survive in and out of the body. They are much larger than viruses and can usually be treated effectively with antibiotics.

BMI — See **Body Mass Index**

Body fluids — Urine, feces, saliva, blood, nasal discharge, eye discharge, and injury or tissue discharge.

Body Mass Index (BMI) — Weight in kilograms divided by height in meters squared. Overweight and obesity can be defined by the BMI for age measurement. Ref: Hagan, J. F., J. S. Shaw, P. M. Duncan. 2008. *Bright futures: Guidelines for health supervision of infants, children and adolescents.* 3rd ed. Elk Grove Village, IL: American Academy of Pediatrics.

Bottle propping — Bottle-feeding an infant by propping the bottle near the infant's mouth and leaving the infant alone rather than holding the bottle by hand.

Botulism — A neuroparalytic disorder characterized by an acute, afebrile, symmetric, descending flaccid paralysis. Paralysis is caused by blockade of neurotransmitter at the voluntary motor and autonomic neuromuscular junctions. Three distinct, naturally occurring forms of human botulism exist: foodborne, wound, and infant. Ref: Pickering, L., ed. 2009. *Red Book: 2009 report of the Committee on Infectious Diseases.* 28th ed. Elk Grove Village, IL: American Academy of Pediatrics.

BPA (BISPHENOL A) — Used to manufacture polycarbonate plastics. This type of plastic is used to make some types of beverage containers, compact disks, plastic dinnerware, impact-resistant safety equipment, automobile parts, and toys. BPA epoxy resins are used in the protective linings of food cans, in dental sealants, and in other products. Ref: Centers for Disease Control and Prevention. 2009. National report on human exposure to environmental chemicals. Fact sheet: Bisphenol A. http://www.cdc.gov/exposurereport/BisphenolA_FactSheet.html.

Care Plan — A document that provides specific health care information, including any medications, procedures, precautions, or adaptations to diet or environment that may be needed to care for a child with chronic medical conditions or special health care needs. Care plans also describe signs and symptoms of impending illness and outline the response needed to those signs and symptoms. A care plan is completed by the primary care provider and should be updated on a regular basis. Ref: Donoghue, E. A., C. A. Kraft, eds. 2010. *Managing chronic health needs in child care and schools: A quick reference guide.* Elk Grove Village, IL: American Academy of Pediatrics.

Caregiver/Teacher — The primary staff who works directly with the children, that is, teacher, aide, or others in a center and the early care and education provider in a small and large family child care home.

Celiac Disease — A digestive disease that damages the small intestine and interferes with absorption of nutrients from food. People who have celiac disease cannot tolerate gluten, a protein in wheat, rye, and barley. Gluten is found mainly in foods but may also be found in everyday products such as medicines, vitamins, and lip balms. Ref: National Digestive Diseases Information Clearinghouse. 2008. Celiac disease. http://digestive.niddk.nih.gov/ddiseases/pubs/celiac/#what.

Child and Adult Care Food Program (CACFP) — The U.S. Department of Agriculture's sponsored program whose early care and education component provides nutritious meals to children enrolled in centers and family child care homes throughout the country.

Child Care Health Consultant — A licensed health professional with education and experience in child and community health and early care and education plus specialized training in child care health consultation.

Child:staff ratio — The amount of staff required, based on the number of children present and the ages of these children.

Children with special health care needs — Children who have or are at increased risk for chronic physical, developmental, behavioral, or emotional conditions who require health and related services of a type or amount beyond that required by children generally. Ref: Maternal and Child Health Bureau. Achieving and Measuring Success: A National Agenda for Children with Special Health Care Needs http://www.mchb.hrsa.gov/programs/specialneeds/achievingsuccess.html.

Chronic — Describing a disease or illness of long duration or frequent recurrence, often having a slow progressive course of indefinite duration. Ref: Merriam-Webster. 2010. Chronic. Medline Plus Medical Dictionary. http://www.merriam-webster.com/medlineplus/chronic.

Clean — To remove dirt and debris by scrubbing and washing with a detergent solution and rinsing with water.

Complementary foods — Solid foods that are age appropriate for infants such as iron-fortified infant cereals and pureed meats.

Compliance — The act of carrying out a recommendation, policy, regulation or procedure.

Contamination — The presence of infectious microorganisms in or on the body, on environmental surfaces, on articles of clothing, or in food or water.

"Cue" feeding — The caregiver/teacher is alert to the infant and child's cues and feeds based on those rather than teach the infant they must "demand" (cry) for their food.

Dental caries — Tooth decay resulting in localized destruction of tooth tissue. Also known as dental cavities.

Diabetes — A group of diseases marked by high levels of blood glucose resulting from defects in insulin production, insulin action, or both. Ref: National Diabetes Education Program. The facts about diabetes: America's seventh leading cause of death. http://www.ndep.nih.gov/diabetes-facts/index.aspx.

Diarrhea — An increased number of abnormally loose stools in comparison with the individual's usual bowel habits.

Disinfect — To destroy or inactivate any germs on any inanimate object.

Dyslipidemia — A condition marked by abnormal concentrations of lipids or lipoproteins in the blood, consisting of one or a combination of high LDL, low HDL, and high triglycerides.

***E. coli* O157:H7** — One of hundreds of strains of Escherichia coli. Although most strains are harmless and live in the intestines of healthy humans and animals, this strain produces a powerful toxin and can cause severe illness, including bloody diarrhea and abdominal cramps. Eating undercooked meat, drinking unpasteurized milk, and swimming in or drinking sewage-contaminated water can cause infection.

Epidemic — Affecting or tending to affect an atypically large number of individuals within a population, community, or region at the same time. Ref: Merriam-Webster. 2010. Epidemic. Medline Plus Medical Dictionary. http://www.merriam-webster.com/medlineplus/epidemic.

EpiPen — An automatic epinephrine injector. Epinephrine is administered in response to some allergic reactions. Ref: Donoghue, E.A., C.A. Kraft, editors.2009. *Managing chronic health needs in child care and schools.* Elk Grove Village, IL: American Academy of Pediatrics.

Ergot — A toxic fungus found as a parasite on grains of rye and other grains. Consumption of food contaminated with ergots may cause vomiting, diarrhea and may lead to gangrene in serious cases. Chronic exposure through consumption of contaminated food can lead to health complications.

Evaluation — Impressions and recommendations formed after a careful appraisal and study.

Facilitated play — To engage children in appropriate play experiences that facilitate development in all domains and promote autonomy, competency and a sense of joy in discovery and learning. Ref: Liske, V., L. Bell. Play and the impaired child. http://www.playworks.net/article-play-and-impaired-child.html

Facility — The buildings, the grounds, the equipment, and the people involved in providing early care and education of any type.

Foodborne illness/disease — An illness or disease transmitted through food products.

Free play — See **Unstructured physical activity**

Galactosemia — A condition in which the body is unable to use (metabolize) the simple sugar galactose. Ref: Medline Plus. 2009. Galactosemia. Medical Encyclopedia. http://www.nlm.nih.gov/medlineplus/ency/article/000366.htm.

Gastric tube feeding — The administration of nourishment through a tube that has been surgically inserted directly into the stomach.

Gross motor skills — Large movements involving the arms, legs, feet, or the entire body (such as crawling, running, and jumping).

Group size — The number of children assigned to a caregiver/teacher or team of caregivers/teachers occupying an individual classroom or well defined space within a larger room. See also Child:Staff Ratio.

Health advocate — In early care and education settings, caregivers/teachers who spend several hours a week with specific duties designed to promote the health and safety of children in their care. They receive special training to prevent, recognize, and correct health and safety problems in early childhood education programs. The health advocate does not fill the same role as the child care health consultant. See also definition for Child Care Health Consultant. Ref: California Childcare Health Program. 2006. *Instructor's guide: The role of the child care health advocate.* University of California, San Francisco School of Nursing, Department of Family Health Care Nursing. http://www.ucsfchildcarehealth.org/pdfs/Curricula/Instuctors_Guide/CCHA_IG_2_Role_v3.pdf

Health care professional — A person who by education, training, certification, or licensure is qualified to and is engaged in providing health care. Ref: http://medical-dictionary.thefreedictionary.com/Health+care+professional

Health consultant — See **Child Care Health Consultant**

Health Plan — See **Care Plan**.

Hepatitis — Inflammation of the liver caused by viral infection. There are six types of infectious hepatitis: type A; type B; nonA, nonB; C; and D.

Human Immunodeficiency Virus (HIV) disease — The virus that can lead to acquired immune deficiency syndrome, or AIDS. HIV damages a person's body by destroying specific blood cells, called CD4+ T cells, which are crucial to helping the body fight diseases. Ref: Centers for Disease Control and Prevention. 2006. HIV/AIDS Basics: What is HIV? http://www.cdc.gov/hiv/resources/qa/definitions.htm.

Hypercholesterolemia — Having elevated cholesterol levels. High levels of cholesterol increase the risk for cardiovascular disease and stroke.

Infant — A child between the time of birth and the age of ambulation (usually the ages from birth through twelve months).

Infection — A condition caused by the multiplication of an infectious agent in the body. Ref: Aronson, S. S., T. R. Shope, eds. 2009. *Managing infectious diseases in child care and schools: A quick reference guide*, 2nd edition. Elk Grove Village, IL: American Academy of Pediatrics.

Ingestion — The act of taking material (whether food or other substances) into the body through the mouth.

Kinesiology — The study of the principles of mechanics and anatomy in relation to human movement. Ref: Merriam-Webster. 2010. Kinesiology. Merriam-Webster Online. http://www.merriam-webster.com/dictionary/kinesiology.

Lecithin — Any of several waxy lipids which are widely distributed in animals and plants, and have emulsifying, wetting, and antioxidant properties.

Lymphoma — A general term for a group of cancers that originate in the lymph system. The two primary types of lymphoma are Hodgkin lymphoma, which spreads in an orderly manner from one group of lymph nodes to another; and non-Hodgkin lymphoma, which spreads through the lymphatic system in a non-orderly manner. Ref: Centers for Disease Control and Prevention. 2009. Hematologic (blood) cancers: Lymphoma. http://www.cdc.gov/cancer/hematologic/lymphoma/.

Medical home — Primary care that is accessible, continuous, comprehensive, family centered, coordinated, compassionate, and culturally effective. The child health care professional/primary care provider works in partnership with the family and patient to ensure that all the medical and non-medical needs of the patient are met. Ref: Hagan, J. F., J. S. Shaw, P. M. Duncan. 2008. *Bright futures: Guidelines for health supervision of infants, children and adolescents.* 3rd ed. Elk Grove Village, IL: American Academy of Pediatrics.

Medications — Any substance that is intended to cure, treat, or prevent disease or is intended to affect the structure or function of the body of humans or other animals.

Morbidity — The incidence of a disease within a population. Ref: Aronson, S. S., T. R. Shope, eds. 2009. *Managing infectious diseases in child care and schools: A quick reference guide*, 2nd edition. Elk Grove Village, IL: American Academy of Pediatrics.

Motor skills — Coordinated muscle movements involved in movement, object control, and postural control perceived as occurring after a stage (or stages) involving birth reflexes, with the idea that fundamental motor skills must be mastered before development of more sport-specific skills. Ref: Barnett, L. M., E. van Beurden, P. J. Morgan, L. O. Brooks, J. R. Beard. 2009. Childhood motor skill proficiency as a predictor of adolescent physical activity. *J Adolescent Health* 44:252–9.

Nasogastric tube feeding — The administration of nourishment using a plastic tube that stretches from the nose to the stomach.

Necrotizing enterocolitis — A condition when the lining of the intestinal wall dies and the tissue falls off. The cause for this disorder is unknown. However, it is thought that a decrease in blood flow to the bowel keeps the bowel from producing mucus that protects the gastrointestinal tract. Bacteria in the intestine may also be a cause. This disorder usually develops in an infant that is already ill or premature, and most often develops while the infant is still in the hospital. Ref: Medline Plus. 2009. Necrotizing enterocolitis. Medical Encyclopedia. http://www.nlm.nih.gov/medlineplus/ency/article/001148.htm.

Nutritionist/Registered Dietitian — A professional with one to two years' experience in infant and child health programs and coursework in child development, who serves as local or state consultant to early care and education staff.

Obesity — Obesity is an excess percentage of body weight (Body Mass Index equal or greater than 95%) due to fat that puts people at risk for many health problems. In children older than two years of age, obesity is assessed by a measure called the Body Mass Index (BMI). Ref: American Academy of Pediatrics. About childhood obesity. http://www.aap.org/obesity/about.html.

Occupational therapy — Treatment based on the engagement in meaningful activities of daily life of a typical child (such as play, feeding, toileting, and dressing). Child specific exercises are developed in order to encourage a child with mental or physical disabilities to contribute to their own recovery and development.

Organisms — Living things. Often used as a general term for germs (such as bacteria, viruses, fungi, or parasites) that can cause disease.

OSHA — Abbreviation for the Occupational Safety and Health Administration of the U.S. Department of Labor, which regulates health and safety in the workplace.

Overweight — Children and adolescents with a BMI equal to or over the 85th percentile for age but less than the 95th percentile for age are considered overweight. Ref: American Academy of Pediatrics. About childhood obesity. http://www.aap.org/obesity/about.html.

Parasite — An organism that lives on or in another living organism (such as ticks, lice, mites).

Parent/Guardian — The child's natural or adoptive mother or father, or other legally responsible person.

Pasteurized — The partial sterilization of a food substance and especially a liquid (as milk) at a temperature and for a period of exposure that destroys objectionable organisms without major chemical alteration of the substance. Ref: Merriam-Webster. 2010. Pasteurization. Merriam-Webster Online. http://www.merriam-webster.com/dictionary/pasteurization.

Perishable Foods — Foods (such as fruit, vegetables, meat, milk and dairy, and eggs) that are liable to spoil or decay. Ref: Merriam-Webster. 2010. Perishable. Merriam-Webster Online. http://www.merriam-webster.com/dictionary/perishable.

Phenylketonuria (PKU) — A genetic disorder in which the body can't process part of a protein called phenylalanine (Phe). Phe is in almost all foods. If the Phe level gets too high, it can damage the brain and cause severe mental retardation. All infants born in U.S. hospitals must now have a screening test for PKU. Ref: National Institute of Child Health and Human Development. 2009. Phenylketonuria. Medline Plus. http://www.nlm.nih.gov/medlineplus/phenylketonuria.html.

Phthalates — A group of chemicals used to make plastics more flexible and harder to break. They are often called plasticizers. They are used in products, such as vinyl, adhesives, detergents, oils, plastics, and personal-care products. Ref: National Report on Human Exposure to Environmental Chemicals. 2009. Fact sheet: Phthalates. Centers for Disease Control and Prevention. http://www.cdc.gov/exposurereport/Phthalates_FactSheet.html.

Physical activity — Any bodily movement produced by the contraction of skeletal muscle that increases energy expenditure above a basal level. Physical activity generally refers to the subset of activity that enhances health. Ref: National Center for Chronic Disease Prevention and Health Promotion. 2008. Physical activity for everyone: Glossary of terms. Centers for Disease Control and Prevention. http://www.cdc.gov/physicalactivity/everyone/glossary/index.html.

Physical therapy — The use of physical agents and methods (such as massage, therapeutic exercises, hydrotherapy, electrotherapy) to assist a child with physical or mental disabilities to optimize their individual physical development or to restore their normal body function after illness or injury.

Pica — A pattern of eating non-food materials (such as dirt or paper). Ref: Medline Plus. 2008. Pica. Medical Encyclopedia. http://www.nlm.nih.gov/medlineplus/ency/article/001538.htm.

Polybrominated diphenyl ethers (PBDE) — Flame-retardant chemicals added to plastics and foam products to make them difficult to burn. Because they are mixed into plastics and foams rather than bound to them, PBDEs can leave the products that contain them and enter the environment. Ref: Agency for Toxic Substances and Disease Registry. 2004. ToxFAQs for Polybrominated diphenyl ethers (PBDEs). http://www.atsdr.cdc.gov/tfacts68-pbde.html.

Preschooler — A child between the age of toilet learning/training and the age of entry into a regular school; usually three to five years of age.

Primary care provider — A person who by education, training, certification, or licensure is qualified to and is engaged in providing health care. A primary care provider coordinates the care of a child with the child's specialist and therapists. Ref: Donoghue, E. A., C. A. Kraft, eds. 2010. *Managing chronic health needs in child care and schools: A quick reference guide.* Elk Grove Village, IL: American Academy of Pediatrics.

Reflux — An abnormal backward flow of stomach contents into the esophagus.

Salmonella — A type of bacteria that causes food poisoning (salmonellosis) with symptoms of vomiting, diarrhea, and abdominal pain.

Salmonellosis — A diarrheal infection caused by Salmonella bacteria.

Sanitize — A process that reduces germs on inanimate surfaces to levels considered safe by public health codes or regulations.

School-age child — This term describes a developmental period associated with a child who is enrolled in a regular school, including kindergarten; usually from five to eighteen years of age. For the purposes of early care and education settings, the maximum age is usually twelve years of age.

Screen time — Time spent watching TV, videotapes, or DVDs; playing video or computer games; and surfing the internet. Ref: Guide to Community Preventive Services. 2010. *Obesity prevention: Behavioral interventions to reduce screen time.* http://www.thecommunityguide.org/obesity/behavioral.html.

Sedentary activity — Non-moving activity like reading, playing a board game, or drawing. Sedentary activity does not provide much physical activity and/or exercise. Ref.: Nemours Health and Prevention Services. 2009. *Best practices for physical activity: A guide to help children grow up healthy — For organizations serving children and youth.* Newark, DE: Nemours Health and Prevention Services. http://www.nemours.org/filebox/service/preventive/nhps/paguidelines.pdf.

SIDS — See **Sudden Infant Death Syndrome**

Staff — Used here to indicate all personnel employed at the facility, including both caregivers/teachers and personnel who do not provide direct care to the children (such as administrators, cooks, drivers, and housekeeping personnel).

Structured physical activity — Caregiver/teacher-led, developmentally appropriate, and fun. Structured activity should include:
- Daily planned physical activity that supports age-appropriate motor skill development. The activity should be engaging and involve all children with minimal or no waiting.
- Daily, fun physical activity that is vigorous (gets children "breathless" or breathing deeper and faster than during typical activities) for short bouts of time.
  Ref: Nemours Health and Prevention Services. 2009. *Best practices for physical activity: A guide to help children grow up healthy — For organizations serving children and youth.* Newark, DE: Nemours Health and Prevention Services. http://www.nemours.org/filebox/service/preventive/nhps/paguidelines.pdf

Sudden Infant Death Syndrome (SIDS) — The sudden death of an infant less than one year of age that cannot be explained after a thorough investigation is conducted, including a complete autopsy, examination of the death scene, and review of the clinical history. Ref: Centers for Disease Control and Prevention. 2009. Sudden Infant Death Syndrome (SIDS) and Sudden Unexpected Infant Death (SUID): Home. http://www.cdc.gov/SIDS/index.htm.

Toddler — A child between the age of ambulation and the age of toilet learning/training, usually thirteen through thirty-five months of age.

Toxoplasmosis — A parasitic disease often causing no symptoms. When symptoms do occur, swollen glands, fatigue, malaise, muscle pain, fluctuating low fever, rash, headache, and sore throat are reported most commonly. Toxoplasmosis can infect and damage a fetus while producing mild or no symptoms in the mother.

Transmission — The passing of an infectious organism or germ from person to person.

Ulcerative colitis — A disease that causes inflammation and sores, called ulcers, in the lining of the rectum and colon. Ulcers form where inflammation has killed the cells that usually line the colon, then bleed and produce pus. Inflammation in the colon also causes the colon to empty frequently, causing diarrhea. Ref: National Institute of Diabetes and Digestive and Kidney Diseases. 2006. Ulcerative colitis. http://digestive.niddk.nih.gov/ddiseases/pubs/colitis/.

Unstructured physical activity — Child-led free play. Unstructured activity should include:
- Activities that respect and encourage children's individual abilities and interests.
- Caregiver/teacher engagement with children, support for extending play, and gentle prompts and encouragement by caregivers/teachers, when appropriate, to stay physically active.
  Ref: Nemours Health and Prevention Services. 2009. *Best practices for physical activity: A guide to help children grow up healthy — For organizations serving children and youth.* Newark, DE: Nemours Health and Prevention Services. http://www.nemours.org/filebox/service/preventive/nhps/paguidelines.pdf

Vegan — Individual does not eat meat, poultry, fish, eggs, or dairy products, only plant foods. Ref: Healthy Children. 2010. Vegetarian diets for children. American Academy of Pediatrics. http://www.healthychildren.org/English/ages-stages/gradeschool/nutrition/Pages/Vegetartian-Diet-for-Children.aspx

Vegetarian — There are various degrees of vegetarianism. Although none eat meat, poultry, or fish, there are other areas in which they vary. Lacto-ovo-vegetarians consume eggs, dairy products, and plant foods and lacto–vegetarians eat dairy products and plant foods but not eggs. Ref: Healthy Children. 2010. Vegetarian diets for children. American Academy of Pediatrics. http://www.healthychildren.org/English/ages-stages/gradeschool/nutrition/Pages/Vegetartian-Diet-for-Children.aspx

Viandas — Root vegetables common in some Hispanic diets. Ref: Block, G., P. Wakimoto, C. Jensen, S. Mandel, R. R. Green. 2006. Validation of a food frequency questionnaire for Hispanics. *Preventing Chronic Disease* 3(3): 1-10. http://www.cdc.gov/pcd/issues/2006/jul/pdf/05_0219.pdf.

Vigorous-intensity physical activity — Rhythmic, repetitive physical activity that uses large muscle groups, causing a child to breathe rapidly and only enabling them to speak in short phrases. Typically children's heart rates are substantially increased and they are likely to be sweating. Ref. Nemours Health and Prevention Services. 2009. *Best practices for physical activity: A guide to help children grow up healthy — For organizations serving children and youth.* Newark, DE: Nemours Health and Prevention Services. http://www.nemours.org/filebox/service/preventive/nhps/paguidelines.pdf

Virus — A microscopic organism, smaller than a bacterium, that may cause disease. Viruses can grow or reproduce only in living cells.

WIC — Abbreviation for the U.S. Department of Agriculture's Special Supplemental Food Program for Women, Infants and Children, which provides food supplements and nutrition education to pregnant and breastfeeding women, infants, and young children who are considered to be at nutritional risk due to their level of income and evidence of inadequate diet.

INDEX